*This book is dedicated
to all those who live with a disability,
to their carers, and to their loved ones.*

Copyright Info

CLARET PRESS

Copyright © Claret Press

The moral right of the authors has been asserted.

Book design by Petya Tsankova

Cover and story illustrations © 2018 Tansy Spinks

tansyspinks.com

ISBN: 978-1-910461-37-2

All rights reserved. No part of this publication may be reproduced, stored in or introduced into a retrieval system, transmitted, in any form, or by any means (electronic, mechanical, photocopying, recording or otherwise) without the prior written consent of the publisher. Any person who does any unauthorised act in relation to this publication may be liable to criminal prosecution and civil claims for damages.

All characters and events in this book, other than those clearly in the public domain, are fictitious and any resemblance to real persons, living or dead, is purely coincidental.

A CIP catalogue record for this book is available from the British Library.

This paperback or can be ordered from all bookstores as well as Amazon.

http://www.claretpress.com

INSIGHTS

Fifteen
Stories
Exploring
Disability

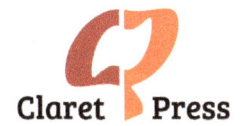

Claret Press

Table of Contents

PREFACE *by Sarah Gray*

DEARBHLA'S BLOUSE *by Nicola Cassidy*	1
DEPRESSION AND THE DENOUEMENT *by Michael Coolwood*	9
BLIND DATE *by Pam Corsie*	23
COLD CALLING *by Claire Goodman*	37
FARMER YOUNG *by Jamie Harding*	41
FOR STEVE *by Jim Knight*	53
HILARY'S FEAST *by Sarah Longthorne*	63
MY SPACESHIP *by Alison McCrossan*	71
FLIGHT *by Roland Miles*	81
FINE NOW *by Diane L. Miller*	85
CARING FOR THE ASTILBIES *by Shirley Muir*	101
HIDDEN IN PLAIN SIGHT *by Bea Mulder*	111
A NEW LEASE OF LIFE *by Neel Patel*	125
ALL I SEE *by Anna Pen*	137
THE TURKEY IN THE BOOT *by Emily White*	145
ABOUT THE CONTRIBUTORS	150
ABOUT THE JUDGES	156

PREFACE *by Sarah Gray*

I'm exhausted. Exhausted to the point that my eyelids droop and I see the room disappear and reappear until only the red interior of my eyelids remains. The gentle rhythm of the ventilator soothes me to the edge of sleep. I'm warm, comfortable and I drop. Wake up! Wake up! Wake up! I have a preface to write. I have a deadline. This is the theme of the collection: carrying on despite living with chronic physical illness, debilitating mental illness, the loss of someone beloved, or the knowledge of imminent death. These stories are intense personal insights into living with complex and challenging conditions. Often humorous, set in faraway places or in futuristic worlds, all are heartfelt and heartbreaking. I thank everyone who entered for sharing their experiences.

Amongst all of these remarkable entries, winners had to be found – an excruciating task given the high standard. Writing short stories is a difficult business at the best of times. We made the competition more challenging by insisting that the stories grapple with a topic too rarely reflected in our literature: mental and physical disability. But we were looking for more than just a nicely constructed story. We wanted innovation, or something quirky, or a spark to amuse or shock. Our top three winners contain all of the necessary ingredients and although their places could easily be swapped, we had to choose.

Winner *For Steve* by Jim Knight is a father and son road trip through backwater USA, ending in a low rent area of Canada. Constructed in two continuous paragraphs, words are used like flashes beyond the car window as it motors through town and country. Only moments, raw and cold, are revealed. At the end of the road lies tragedy and redemption.

Written with humour and a delicate touch, our second place winner, *Fine Now* by Diane Miller, has a classic structure containing an unusual tale. Isolated by her disease and her family's misunderstanding of it, Ellen suffers alone. Living in despair, Ellen is hopeless and lonely until an unwelcome addition to the family provides her with the understanding she craves.

And our final choice is *Blind Date* by Pam Corsie. This marvellous tale is a reminder that people are more than their disability. Despite the characters' perceived impediments to love, both James (a portly physique) and Annabelle (impaired vision) are determined to find 'the one'. The tension is palpable. All you need is love and that is true for everybody.

I'm exhausted. Exhausted but satisfied, I allow my eyelids to droop, the room disappears and reappears until only the red interior of my eyelids remain. The ventilator gently soothes me to the edge sleep. I'm warm, comfortable and I drop. In my sleep, I dream, my stories evolve, taking shape, characters live and meaning emerges. When I wake, I'm ready to carry on. I am ready to write.

Our third judge, Dr James Scott, deserves thanks for giving his professional opinion. He made me think more closely about my choices and the reasons I made them. Thank you. I also have to thank Katie Isbester, Editor-in-Chief at Claret Press, for choosing to use my stories as the inspiration for this competition and asking me to co-judge. I'm flattered and humbled. Thank you to the team at Claret Press, Anastasia Antonova, Sanne Steele-Nicholson, Suzanne Verheul, Philippa Gould, Isobelle Lans and Joshua Hunter, for all their hard work in coordinating the competition and producing such an impressive collection. The collection has been made all the more beautiful as celebrated artist Tansy Spinks has donated her wonderful photographs. Thank you, Tansy.

These stories resonate with our shared humanity. Charities research, inform, and care for those with disability. Charities act on our deepest humanitarian responses and for our shared humanity. The net proceeds from the sale of this book are going to support the Motor Neuron Disease Association, which helps people like me. Join me in supporting its essential work, with our thanks.

Sarah Gray
October 2018

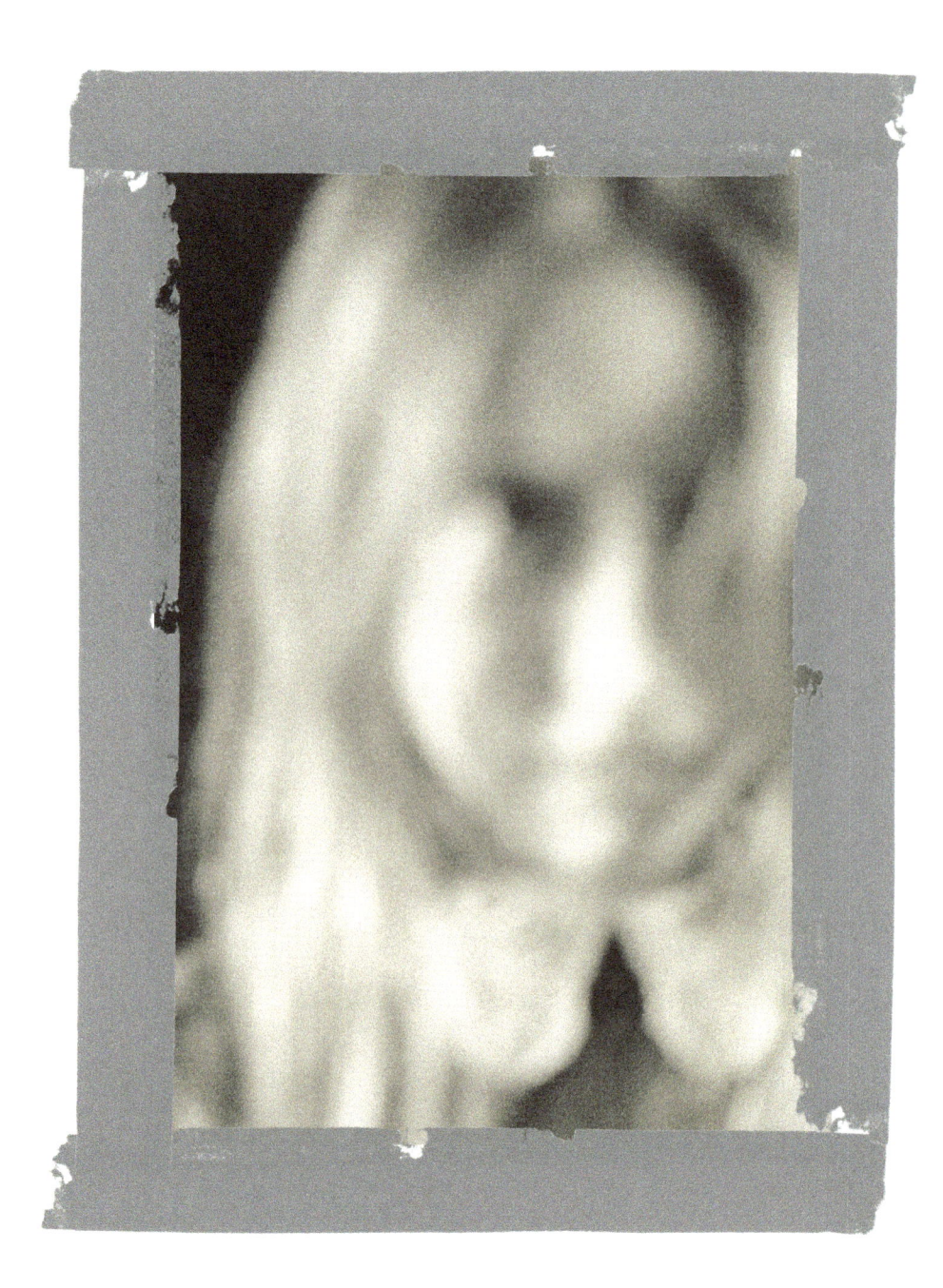

DEARBHLA'S BLOUSE

by Nicola Cassidy

I'd like to say she looked the same. But she doesn't. Does anyone ever really, in the coffin? Do you think that's just something people say – to give comfort? *Doesn't she look lovely, just like she's sleeping*? Only she's not sleeping.

She's gone.

That's what my mother had said to me when she told me. 'She's gone.'

Gone where? I'd thought. Gone in, because that had happened before? Stolen on a summer's day, the sun perched high behind wispy, cirrus clouds. Looking down on the horror. A grief we were all part of.

But she hadn't gone in, not this time. This time it was too late. This time, she had gone beyond, too far, away from us. It was over.

We had let her down.

I know that.

I stare at Dearbhla's neck, tucked into a pristine blouse. The blouse is pearl white, silk, the buttons covered in a material a slightly different shade. Maybe it's the glue that changed the colour, from pearl white to off white?

This wasn't the outfit I'd picked out. I'd chosen a dress, a blue one, material that showed off her eyes, the sparkle in them.

But of course, her eyes were closed. And the sparkle had been cleaned away.

Still, where is the dress? Why this high-necked blouse, a blouse I recognize?

A flicker of anger fidgets my head. I touch my forehead, this is too much.

'Doesn't she look lovely?' says Cheryl.

I don't respond.

'Just like she's sleeping,' she says.

I listen to Cheryl's dramatic sigh.

Cheryl barely knew Dearbhla and, as is her habit, would have had nothing good to say about her anyway. *Suffers with her nerves*, Cheryl would have said. *Been in and out of Kilmanny you know.*

Cheryl is enjoying the drama of all of this.

So young. Her whole life ahead of her.

Yes, but what sort of life?

'I was reading about electric shock treatment,' Mam had said one day, a *Woman's Own* in her hand.

I looked at her over my cereal, the spoon hovering at my mouth.

'In *Woman's Own*?'

'No!' said Mam. 'It was in the paper the other day. It resets the brainwaves. You know, like a kickstart.'

I'd snorted. A cornflake had blown from my spoon and fluttered clumsily back into the bowl. I'd put the spoon down.

'I don't think so, Mam.'

'Well I'm just talking out loud. That medication doesn't seem to be working.'

She'd thrown her eyes up to the ceiling, towards Dearbhla's bedroom. She'd been in there maybe two weeks at that stage, curled up in the bed, like a cat waiting to kitten. Crying. Sleeping. Blackouts.

I'd brought trays to the door, knocked, gone in to the fetid, dim dark. She'd turned over in the bed, hunched, and I'd looked at her face, trying to get her to look at me. It was always futile, she couldn't, and I'd realise that I didn't recognise her.

Her skin had changed, the melancholy melting her features, morphing her bright eyes and porcelain skin into something smudged, almost wiped away.

In those episodes, her spirit had left her, upping and floating, out the skylight perhaps, towards the tips of the trees, disappearing like the parrot helium balloon we'd let go of when we were small and watched, in flight, into the sky, free.

I'd soothed, talking gently, brightly, my words a mask of the anguish I felt. I would get her through this. I would get her the help she needed. She had so much to look forward to.

'You did everything you could,' says Cheryl, staring at Dearbhla's waxy brow.

How would she know that? How would Cheryl know what we did?

I nod my head in some sort of answer, an automatic response I've been giving non-stop to my fellow mourners for the past four days now.

She's in shock, I hear them whisper. *She's taking it very bad.*

Cheryl knows nothing of the everything I did, all those web pages and forums visited, doctors, psychiatrists, consultants, clinicians. Deep depression, clinical depression, schizophrenia, bi-polar. Borderline Personality Disorder.

Searching for a label, for a name, for an answer.

It was I who had her taken her to Kilmanny that day, that scorching, shimmering summer's day, walking with her, my arm linked in hers, supporting, as she'd struggled to walk. The building had loomed down upon us, its grey façade not so imposing up close.

The thought of it had been worse than the reality.

We'd waited in a small, beige room, anticipating the doctor who would come, the miracle he would work.

She couldn't promise not to harm herself.

And so in she went; it was their policy.

Committed.

I look at Dearbhla's hands, clasped in prayer around a set of rosary beads, black, pieced together by silver metal, the cross hanging across her bony fingers. Her nails are painted a light pink, but I can see the blue coming through, as though they are bruised.

Mam must have gotten the rosary beads. Dearbhla would be raging, she hated religion, had left the church years ago as a teenager. I think about wrenching them from her clenched hands, tossing them out the open sitting room window, left wide to circulate the air in this stuffy funeral room.

But it would upset Mam. And I wasn't sure if I'd be able to prise the fingers.

'Would you like a cup of tea?' asks Cheryl.

I shake my head.

My stomach is a knot, twisted, nothing going in or out. I cannot eat. I can't imagine ever eating again. I know I have shed weight already, maybe half a stone.

Cheryl's hand is on my back. I want to shake it off like a flea. Instead, I stay, rooted, staring, back to Dearbhla's blouse.

They've curled her hair, lightly, it falls, lovely, down her shoulders, around the silk.

I was always envious of her deep chestnut hair. It ran down her back like a carpet and when it got really long, Mam would take the big kitchen scissors to it and snip it across the back, snip snip snip. I loved the sound of those scissors as they severed the hair, watching the clumps and fleck falling onto an outlay of newspaper on the floor.

When she was fifteen, she'd cut it up short, spiky for a while, like a boy, Mam said. She'd dyed it different colours, bleaching it and steeping it, orange, grape, deep chalky black. Last year she shaved part of it, all around the front, it felt good, she said.

Now the shaved part was a fringe. A forever fringe. No more dye jobs or hatchet jobs or expressing herself through her razor cut.

Cheryl moves off, unnerved by my silence, by my stony face and lack of words. I care not. I care nothing, for no one. I cared for Dearbhla and what good did that do?

The medication can take some time to work, the community nurse had said the last time she'd called to check on her, a new system, a system where Dearbhla needn't go in anymore.

They came to you. Loonies on wheels. Ding dong doorstep.

I reach out and touch the rigid collar of the blouse, feeling its cool, satin texture. My fingertips edge over the tiny ruffles.

And then I remember. The blouse.

It's mine, it's not Dearbhla's at all.

I wore it to an interview, some years back, an admin job, front desk, reception, looking presentable.

Mam is beside me, she does this, leading people up to the coffin, telling them to look at Dearbhla, smiling manically and they all say the same thing.

She looks just like she's sleeping.

'The blouse,' I say to Mam. 'That's mine.'

'What?' says Mam.

'It's mine.'

'What are you talking about?'

Her eyes are ringed red, mascara long gone, dark smudges under her eyes, like shadows.

Tears sting the back of my eyes.

'Where's the dress, the blue one, I picked it out?'

'Darling…' Mam says.

She looks at Dearbhla. Then back to me.

'Darling, her neck.'

The rope. Wiry and rough, choking, bruised.

The blouse is high necked. One of the only high-necked garments between our wardrobes.

Mam's hand is on my back, rubbing lightly between the shoulder blades. She doesn't say anything. What is there to say?

The man standing beside Mam is a neighbour. Pat is his name. He smells of weed killer.

'Looks just like she's sleeping, doesn't she?' he says, bowing his head.

I can feel the words, bubbling, in my throat.

Mam tenses, sensing perhaps the outburst. She can always tell when it was coming. I feel her hand stiffen on my back.

'No!' I roar. 'She doesn't look like she's sleeping. She's not sleeping. She's fucking dead!'

The wave of silence washes over the room, conversations interrupted, low mumbling arrested. Someone clinks a coffee cup.

My shoulders are heaving, water streaming down my face.

Mam has her arm around my shoulder, telling me to shush.

Pat looks mortified.

She leads me away and I let the tears fall, not even wiping them away.

Mam wants me to lie down.

You're overcome.

I go to Dearbhla's bed, the bed that bore her days, weeks, and months of tears.

'Why couldn't we save her Mam?' I say, as she folds me into the bed, my eyes wet, my nose a river.

'She couldn't save herself,' Mam says.

She pats me on the forehead and I realise in that moment, how much I love mother, how strong she is, how she has borne this torment before I even knew what it was. I have lost a sister, but she has lost much more than that.

In the dusk, the yellow light filtering through the skylight frames particles that swirl and rise in the air. I look at them dashing and flicking, rising and falling, magic dust.

As my eyes adjust, I see a hanger, coming into focus, hung from the top of the tall mirror in the corner of Dearbhla's room.

The blue dress.

You can take a lend of it if you like.

I hear her voice, soft, cheerful, like before.

I'll swap my blouse for your dress.

Okay then.

Okay then.

I will wear it to the funeral.

In honour.

I close my eyes after Mam leaves and hear the murmur from below.

Mourners, moving, coming and going, drinking tea and coffee, eating cake.

Looking at Dearbhla, with her fringe and her blouse.

Sleeping.

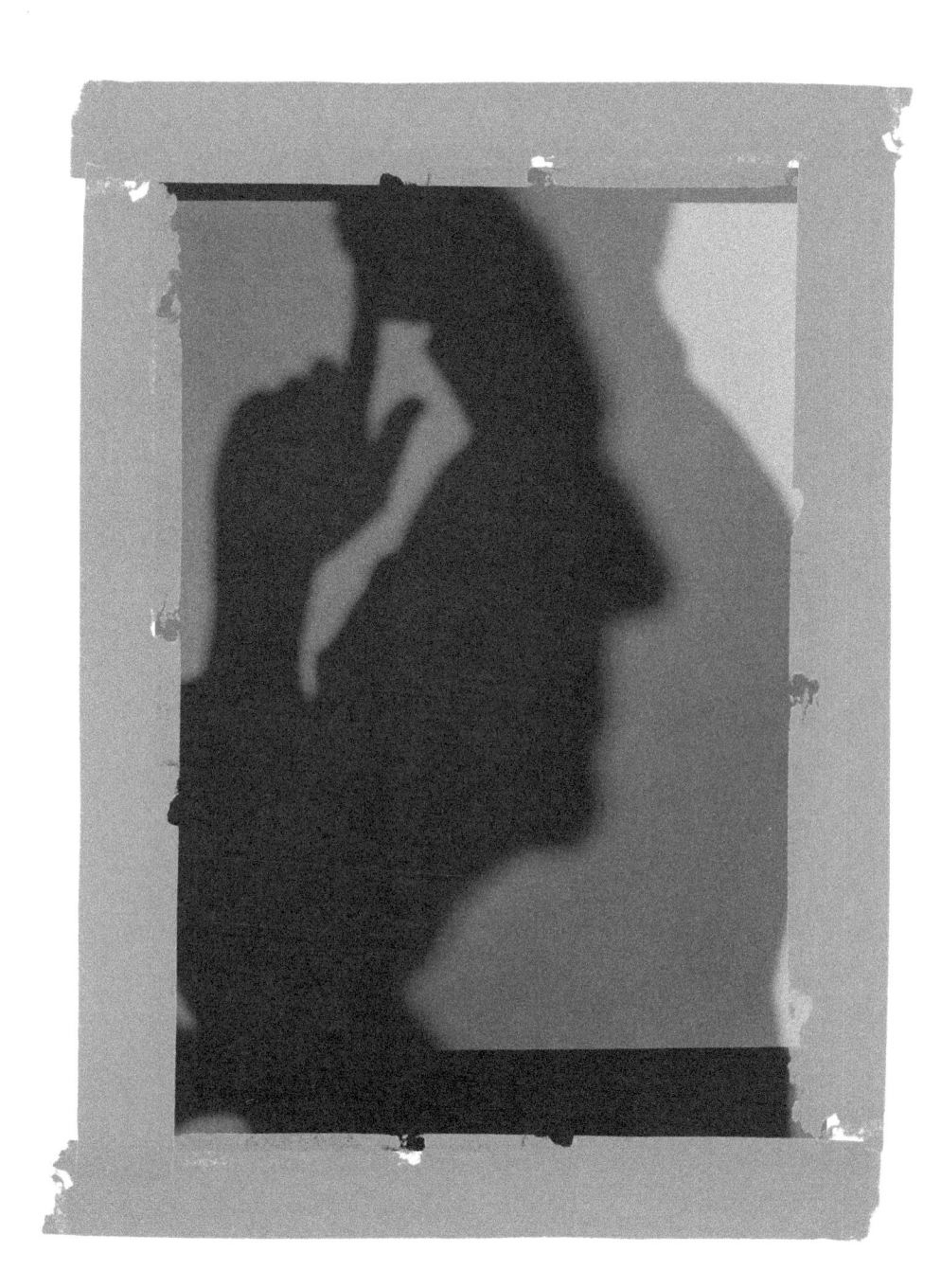

DEPRESSION AND THE DENOUEMENT

by Michael Coolwood

'This case has been most singular from the start!' declared Inspector Tamworth. She began to pace the length of the living room. Her suspects were arranged in front of her whilst her trusty constable guarded the door to ensure there was no escape.

'Ryousuke Tenya, heir to the Tenya family estate, was found dead on the ground outside this very house yesterday evening. His neck was broken and there was a strip of cloth clutched in his hand. That cloth belonged to Alistair Gus, the only child of trade magnate Maria Gus. Alistair had no alibi, so he was held by the families until I could arrive.'

Inspector Tamworth rounded on her constable. 'Constable! What did I say as soon as I cast my eyes over the crime scene?'

Constable Depression opened her notebook and flicked to the appropriate page. 'You said that you couldn't work out which idea was worse: That you'd die alone or that you'd find someone who loved you and you'd then proceed to make them as miserable as you are.'

'Exactly!' cried Inspector Tamworth. 'Exactly,' she repeated. She started to chew her fingernails.

'Sorry,' said Beckett, who was acting as security for the house party, 'what has that got to do with the case?'

Tamworth glanced at Depression, who mouthed the word 'everything'.

'It has everything to do with everything!' Tamworth replied. 'How can I live with myself if I know that my very presence drags the mood of others down to my level?'

The suspects exchanged glances.

'But specifically the case of the murder of Ryousuke Tenya,' Beckett prompted.

Tamworth suddenly focussed. 'Yes, of course, you're right. It has nothing to do with the case, does it Depression?'

'No, ma'am,' replied Depression. 'You shouldn't have brought it up.'

'Quite right, Depression. I really am unbelievably stupid sometimes,' nodded Tamworth thoughtfully. 'Returning to the case, then, it seemed remarkable that Alistair had the strength to snap Ryousuke Tenya's neck, so I searched for other methods by which the eldest child of House Tenya might have met his fate. There was one obvious answer!'

'Quite right, ma'am!' Depression interjected. 'No one ever wants to spend time with you socially, your only human contact is when you have to investigate a murder. People have to literally die before anyone will agree to talk to you.'

'No, no,' Tamworth tutted, waving an impatient hand at Depression. 'Well, not "no", quite obviously that's true, but I meant Ryousuke Tenya must have fallen from a window or the roof, breaking his neck due to the fall.'

'Very good, ma'am,' murmured Depression. 'But it's wise to keep focus on that other matter as well.'

'Kindly make a note of it,' nodded Tamworth.

Depression drew out a pencil, blacker than night, and began to scrawl incomprehensible squiggles on her notebook.

'Sorry,' Beckett interjected, 'why is she here?'

'Who?' Tamworth asked, focusing on Beckett.

'Depression. Why is she here? It doesn't seem like she's helping much.'

'Ah!' Tamworth cried, snapping her fingers. 'I can't get rid of her. I tried once or twice – I had some therapy, standard sort of stuff, but whatever I try she always seems to come back, so I've just decided to... er... to... what was it I decided to do, Depression?'

'You decided to give up and let me control every aspect of your life, ma'am,' oozed Depression. 'There's no point in trying to overcome me, you'll never get better. It's futile even to try.'

Tamworth turned back to Beckett with a 'does that answer your question' expression.

Beckett blinked. 'I don't think that's true, Inspector. I haven't known you long but you seem to be clever and pleasant company, it seems that Depression is just lying to you.'

Tamworth frowned. She turned to Depression, who shook her head. Tamworth turned back to Beckett. 'Well, I'll consider what you say of course,' she lied. 'But I should really get on with explaining the course of events that led up to the fire. You see, Depression and I checked the rooms over when Ryousuke Tenya's body was found. There were no signs of a struggle and it was doubtful that a fall from these windows would have been lethal. The blood that was found at the scene left it unlikely that Ryousuke Tenya's body had been moved. This left only one option. The roof!'

Depression sidled forwards and whispered in Inspector Tamworth's ear. Tamworth nodded. 'Just so,' she frowned. 'There were, in fact, two options. The first was that I do not deserve to be healthy. I should try to feel better by indulging in the stash of biscuits I keep in my car because whilst I know they will not help in the long term; they will make me feel better in this moment. The other option was... the roof!

'I therefore attempted to gain access to the roof but found the door locked. After I made a quick stop at my car to retrieve my biscuit supply, I attempted to locate the key. I was informed that only two people had a key to the roof: Ryousuke Tenya and his mother, Hisako Tenya. Now, Hisako had been spotted arguing with her son the previous evening but she was very composed when I interviewed her. Depression mentioned that she might just not want to interact with me in any way, much like my friends and family, but I dismissed this thought after considering it for ten minutes or so.

'I enquired as to the whereabouts of Hisako Tenya's key to the roof. She searched for it and reported that it was missing. She noted that this was unusual. Depression and I checked for Ryousuke Tenya's key and likewise found it missing. One missing key could be a coincidence. Two missing keys is a clue!'

'Did Depression really help you search?' Beckett asked. 'She doesn't seem particularly helpful.'

'Well I say "helped",' Tamworth nodded. 'It wasn't exactly help. She forced me to sit in my car for three hours, unable to do anything but stare out of the window and reflect on how awful I am.'

'That's not true, Inspector!' Beckett cried. 'I'm sure you're not awful!'

'Well of course I know that,' snapped Tamworth. 'On an intellectual level I know that, but on the other hand, when you think about it, it's definitely true.'

'It really isn't,' Beckett objected.

'Agreed!' chimed in Alistair. 'You've spent the last twelve hours trying to prove I'm not a murderer. That's not an awful thing to do!'

Tamworth narrowed her eyes. She glanced at Depression, who shrugged. 'Well, maybe,' she admitted, 'but maybe you are, in fact, the murderer, Alistair!'

'Oh come on, we've all worked out that Alistair isn't the murderer by now.' Beckett scoffed.

'Have we?' asked Duchess Lenora Mountbatten, who had been quiet up to that moment. There was a round of conformations from the other suspects. Duchess Lenora looked a little worried.

'So, I began to search for the missing keys whilst Depression reminded me of how lazy I am. I should have solved the case by now. Why hadn't I solved it? I clearly didn't actually want to solve it. I was a burden on everyone around me.'

'Inspector, I feel like we should be getting you some help,' interjected Beckett.

'In a minute, in a minute, I'm getting to the good bit,' said Tamworth. 'You see, I eventually found the keys. They had been buried in a flowerbed. A patch of recently disturbed soil betrayed their resting place. This was most curious, most curious indeed. Why go to the trouble of hiding the keys to the roof? Clearly there was something up there that the murderer did not want Depression or me to see!

'To recap the crime for those who haven't been paying attention, the body was found at 8pm. Duchess Lenora Mountbatten kindly provided us with a photograph taken of her with the victim at 7pm, meaning he was most certainly alive at that time. Before that, Alistair reported an item missing – a brooch that he was to wear during the ceremonial reading of friendship between people that was to happen that evening.'

'Is that strictly relevant?' Beckett asked.

'Oh it may well be,' Tamworth smiled. 'So, after 7pm, we can account for the movements of Duchess Lenora Mountbatten in their entirety but there are times when everyone else could have slipped off to murder Ryousuke Tenya. Thus, we must turn our attention to motive.'

At this, Constable Depression coughed. 'Ma'am,' she interrupted. 'You wanted me to remind you that everyone is judging you for your tearfulness, low mood and lack of ability to socialise. You should be hiding in your bedroom.'

'Yes, all right, Depression, give it a rest,' Tamworth grinned. 'I'm in the middle of my flow here.'

Depression looked worried at this development. She started flicking through her notebook and soon found what she was looking for. She stabbed a finger at a page and opened her mouth to speak. Tamworth did not give her the chance.

'The reason I do not believe Alistair murdered Ryousuke Tenya is that the two had only just met. Yes, they had argued, but these disagreements had not been particularly vindictive. It seemed merely a clash of personalities. Alistair was a model student and had no previous arrests or cautions for violent behaviour. His mother, Maria, has some slight question marks hanging over her past, but this is not something we should tar Alistair with.

'Might Maria have chosen to avenge herself on Ryousuke Tenya for the arguments between Alistair and the victim? Possibly, but there are two problems with this line of thought: First, Alistair is a teenage boy. If his mother wished to avenge every slight or argument, then she must get up very early in the morning indeed to arrange that many deaths. Secondly, if it was Maria who actually committed the murder, why was evidence linking the crime to Alistair found at the scene?'

'You're going on a bit, ma'am,' Depression hissed. 'I'm duty bound to remind you that when you go on a bit, people find you boring.

Particularly your relationship with me. People don't like that you keep bringing it up and that's why no one wants to spend time with you.'

Tamworth rounded on Depression and raised a finger. She opened her mouth but then paused. 'Fair point,' she nodded. She stared down at her shoes. 'Fair point indeed.'

Silence reigned for a time.

Tamworth looked around. She found an empty chair. She collapsed into it with a sigh.

'Are you okay, Inspector?' Alistair asked. His mum rested a hand on his shoulder and he looked up into her eyes, confused.

'Yes, thank you, I'm fine,' Tamworth lied. 'I just need a minute.'

Tamworth pinched the bridge of her nose and squeezed her eyes shut. Wetness glistened at the corners of her eyes.

'Other motives,' she muttered, eventually, 'consist of some work Beckett did for the victim. Maybe there was something Beckett uncovered that led to the victim's death. It seems to be a stretch, particularly as we found a more compelling motive in the papers that Beckett passed over to the victim. We also found some irregularities in Hisako Tenya's business dealings.'

'Did you indeed?' Hisako Tenya asked, sitting up a little straighter in her chair.

'Yup,' nodded Tamworth, apparently not having the energy to stand back up yet. 'Why don't you tell us all about that?'

Hisako sighed. 'Ryousuke came to me with some scurrilous accusations.'

'About?' Tamworth asked.

'About some irregularities in my company's pension fund.'

Tamworth nodded. 'Go on.'

'We discussed the matter and we mutually decided that I should retire as soon as possible and donate some of my personal finances to the company I helped grow so as to stabilise it a little.'

'You mean you were embezzling and Ryousuke Tenya made you give the money back and take early retirement?' Tamworth asked. She still didn't appear able to take her eyes off her shoes.

'Well I wouldn't put it quite like that...' Hisako stated.

DEPRESSION AND THE DENOUEMENT

'No doubt, but I have copies of the documents that Ryousuke Tenya confronted you with. No doubt you will be able to provide some proof of your intent to take early retirement?'

'I sent a letter to my lawyer, she should have it by now.'

'Very good,' Tamworth said. She slapped her thighs and stood, groaning slightly.

'This just leaves Duchess Lenora Mountbatten. You don't have a motive, do you, Duchess?'

All eyes turned to the Duchess. She shook her head, regally.

Tamworth groaned.

'Ma'am, you're making a meal out of your condition again,' Depression stated, coldly. 'You know people hate it when you are selfishly having a difficult time in front of them.'

Tamworth wobbled slightly. 'Agreed. So now,' she said, 'we need to talk about the fire. Someone set a fire in Ryousuke Tenya's office. No one was hurt but most of his paperwork was destroyed. Clearly whoever set this wanted to destroy some evidence. It might have been Hisako Tenya but then, Hisako, you knew that your son had entrusted some documents to you before his death, didn't you?'

Hisako nodded.

'I'm sorry,' Duchess Lenora Mountbatten coughed. 'He did what?'

'Yes, I thought you might be a little surprised by that news,' Tamworth grinned. A little spark appeared to be creeping back into her gaze. 'Yes, Ryousuke Tenya was a cautious individual. He liked to keep copies of his documents and, knowing how much emphasis his mother put on the importance of trust and family, he entrusted the documents to her. These documents also included the evidence of her embezzling from the pension fund.'

Hisako was struck by a coughing fit at that moment.

'My apologies,' Tamworth nodded, 'embezzling is such an ugly word. Let us leave it at "Hisako's unauthorised deflation of the pension fund." This deflation is, coincidentally, another point in Hisako's favour. If she had murdered Ryousuke in order to cover up her actions, she would scarcely have kept his document stash in her office, given the stash concealed evidence of her guilt.'

'What else did the document stash contain?' Duchess Lenora Mountbatten asked, casually.

The forced jollity of her voice caused everyone in the room to look at her, even Constable Depression, who had been busy whispering dark sentences into the ear of Inspector Tamworth.

'Nothing much on the face of it,' Tamworth smiled. 'Certainly nothing too shocking to most in this room. You have a secret child, Duchess Lenora. Ryousuke had made a note that he wanted to meet them.'

Hisako looked shocked by this news, no one else in the room seemed to care much. Duchess Lenora did her best to look unconcerned by this revelation. Inspector Tamworth passed her gaze over the suspects, one by one, before shrugging.

'Well, maybe it was nothing,' she remarked. 'But it gives you a motive for murder, Duchess Lenora, does it not? The Tenya family are extremely traditional. Ryousuke Tenya would have been unwilling to do business with you without meeting your child and you wished to prevent that, to keep your secret safe. You could very well have murdered him to prevent that.'

'I could, yes, I could,' the Duchess replied. 'But I also could not have.'

Tamworth waited to see if there was a follow up. 'Compelling,' she nodded, when it became clear that there wasn't going to be one.

'I didn't want to risk incriminating myself,' the Duchess explained.

'Very sensible.'

'Just in case you don't actually know who did the murder.'

'Oh no, I understand, your prudence is commendable.'

'I think I might still get away with this, so I don't want to ruin it by opening my big mouth.'

'I understand completely,' the inspector intoned. 'So, moving right along to your alibi, Duchess.'

'Could I just remind you, ma'am, that you're a failure of a human being?' interrupted Depression.

'Yes, thank you, Depression, I'll get to that in a minute. Now, Duchess, could you explain your alibi to me? I'm having a little trouble with it.'

The Duchess shifted about in her chair. 'What's to explain?' she asked. 'It's a picture. It shows me and the victim, very much alive, at 7pm.

What's the problem? What's the problem? I don't understand? What's the problem?'

'Maybe I just need a fresh pair of eyes on the photograph in question,' Tamworth mused. She handed it to Alistair. 'Could you tell me what you see, Alistair?'

Alistair took a thickly-rimmed pair of glasses out of a pocket and slipped them on. 'It's the victim and Duchess Lenora,' he reported. 'They're in the living room of this house. There's a clock in the background and, yes, it says 7pm. Only the 12 and the 6 are marked on the clock but the hour hand is pointing at where the seven would be if the clock was less pretentious.'

Tamworth nodded. Constable Depression whispered into her ear but the Inspector swatted her colleague away. 'Tell me, did anyone in this room take this photograph?'

The suspects looked at each other. No one volunteered themselves as the mysterious photographer.

'Duchess, do you remember who took the photograph?'

Duchess Lenora paused for a second too long before answering. 'Actually, no one took the photograph. We used a self-timer on the camera.'

Tamworth nodded. 'Interesting. Why do that when you could have got any of these people here to take the picture for you, or a servant?'

'I don't know. Just a whim. Shut up. It's a perfectly normal thing to do.'

'Just so. Well then, may I ask why you chose to stand where you stood?'

'I believe Ryousuke Tenya selected that position.'

'I don't believe you.'

'Don't you?'

'No.'

'That's a pity.'

'Isn't it?' Tamworth smiled, thinly. 'You see, I knew something was wrong with this photograph when I first saw it. I spent some time in the living room just now and when I saw what was wrong, the method of the crime and the person behind it was suddenly obvious.'

'It was, was it?' the Duchess asked.

'Yes.'

'Damn.'

'Just so. You see, the living room of this house boasts a mirror. It is not particularly large as these things go, but then this photograph is framed strangely. We only see two thirds of each subject and they are posed awkwardly in order to ensure the clock is in shot. That is not suspicious in itself. What is suspicious, however, is that everything in the picture is mirrored. It is almost as if person who chose the location of this photograph chose to shoot its subjects in a mirror whilst making sure to get a clock in shot but not the camera.'

'Ah, no, you see,' blurted the Duchess, 'no, because, because, well, because if it was a mirror, then I would be holding my newspaper in my left hand, whereas you can clearly see in that picture that it's in my right hand.'

'She's got you there, ma'am,' Depression moaned.

'Oh leave it alone, Depression, it's obvious that she just held her newspaper in her other hand for the purposes of creating an alibi. You really are just trying to get in my way, aren't you?'

'That's right, ma'am.' Depression nodded. She sniffed dejectedly and started to pick at her fingernails.

'You've ruined what I was going to say next anyway, Depression. I was going to do this terribly clever thing where I pretended to believe her and then ask an innocent question that torpedoed her excuse amidships.'

'Sorry, ma'am, I didn't mean to spoil your fun,' lied Depression. 'You could still give the line a go, maybe, but do be aware that everyone is staring at you and they'd probably think you were insufferably smug if you tried doing it now, especially given I've now drawn attention to the awkwardness.'

'Look, Inspector, we're all very impressed by your handling of the case so far, we're agog to hear the rest of your explanation,' urged Beckett, trying to wrestle control of the conversation back away from Constable Depression.

'Thank you, Beckett, that means a lot,' Tamworth smiled, gravely.

'Many of my suspects aren't nearly so patient and supportive as you all have been today.'

'Indeed!' yelped the Duchess, shooting to her feet. 'In fact, I propose that we allow the Inspector a brief moment to collect herself so she can resume her explanation in the manner she is accustomed to. Now, since we've all agreed to do that, would you all please excuse me for a moment? I have a pressing need to escape – no. I have a pressing need to flee – no. What's a better way to put this? I need to run aw... no.'

Everyone gave the Duchess a few moments to think about her choice of words. Alistair offered to go up to his room to fetch his thesaurus for her. The Duchess politely declined.

'I need,' the Duchess concluded after nodding to herself, 'to saunter away in a not-remotely-suspicious manner, to a place that is none of your concern but might well be located in Switzerland.'

Inspector Tamworth gave the Duchess ten seconds of silence in case she wanted to improve on this excuse a little. It became clear that she didn't when the aristocrat rose regally from her armchair and started trying to sidle around Constable Depression.

'I'm sorry, Duchess, but Constable Depression is absolutely inescapable. Even if you somehow got past her and out of the door, you would find her trailing you everywhere you went. Believe me, the constable has been with me for fifteen years at this point. I can never escape her; all I can do is learn to live with her. I have developed strategies that enable me to cope with her worst excesses thanks to therapy and medication.'

'Are you saying that if I have therapy and medication that Constable Depression will let me go?' the Duchess asked, hopefully. She made another unsuccessful attempt to dodge around the stolid constable.

'No, that is very much not what I said,' sighed Tamworth. 'Duchess, do come and sit back down, you'll want to know how I have pierced your alibi.'

'Oh, go on then,' the Duchess groaned as she sulked back to her armchair.

'You see, Duchess, you – or whoever it is that arranged for this photograph, but to be clear it was most definitely you – forgot one crucial fact about mirrors.'

'Ooh! Is it that everything in a reflection appears reversed?' Alistair asked.

'Very good, Alistair!' Tamworth beamed. 'As you will note from the photograph, not only are the numbers on the clock mirrored, but the hands on the clock are mirrored as well, meaning we have for all this time been misinterpreting the time they were pointing to! To put it another way, your alibi is not, in fact, for 7pm! It is for 5pm!'

Everyone in the room gasped appreciatively, except for Constable Depression, who gasped sarcastically, and the Duchess, who gasped begrudgingly.

'But what does that have to do with the actual facts of the case?' Beckett asked. 'After all, it was a scrap of Alistair's clothing that was found in the victim's hand and it was a brooch of Alistair's that was found on the roof which the victim was pushed from. Why are you spending so much time trying to bust the Duchess's alibi?'

'She's got y–'

'No she has not "got me there", Depression, shut up. Thank you for your point, Beckett, but the facts of the case mean that Alistair is the one person who could not be the murderer. You see, if Alistair was so careless as to leave two key pieces of evidence behind on the victim's body and at the crime scene, why would he take the time to lock the door to the roof and hide they key to the lock, rather than simply removing the evidence from the roof?'

'Well...' began Duchess Lenora, tentatively.

'No, Duchess, you are wrong. In fact, the most likely course of events is as follows: The murder took place sometime shortly after 5pm. Certain items of Alistair's were procured beforehand and then planted to throw suspicion onto him. One of these items was reported missing at 6pm. It was therefore imperative to secure the crime scene and prevent anyone at all from accessing the roof.'

'But why?' Beckett asked.

'You –' began Depression.

'Shut up, Depression,' snapped Tamworth. 'The crime scene needed to be secured, because if Alistair's missing item had been left there before 6pm, then the victim had already been murdered by that point. This means that Duchess Lenora's alibi is clearly a false one, given that it appears to show the victim alive at 7pm. In order for Duchess Lenora to preserve her alibi – I meant to say 'the murderer' just then but I may as well stop pretending – hang on… let me start again. In order for Duchess Lenora to preserve her alibi, she needed to prevent us from discovering these details.

'So, with that in mind, Duchess Lenora has the motive, means and opportunity. She has no alibi. Duchess, I submit that you are the guilty party. Do you have anything to say? Any neat little confessions? No? Are you going to do a little speech?'

Duchess Lenora looked furtive. 'Sorry,' she said. 'I honestly didn't think I would get caught so I didn't give any thought to this eventuality.'

'Fair enough,' nodded Tamworth, 'Forget I said anything, Duchess. If I were you I'd keep my mouth shut until your lawyer gets here.'

'But she basically confessed in front of all of us,' objected Alistair. 'Surely she won't get away with it after doing something so stupid?'

'It depends how bribeable her jury is, really,' shrugged Tamworth. 'Anyway, another case solved, Constable Depression!'

'Right you are, ma'am. Shall we return to the station to write up our reports and then we can spend the evening exploring an unhealthy relationship with alcohol? It will make you feel better in the short term!'

'No, no.' Tamworth mused, 'I think I'll go for a run.'

'Oh, I wouldn't do that, ma'am,' Depression objected, as Tamworth strode from the room.

'Isn't she going to arrest me?' the Duchess asked.

'Damn!' cried Tamworth, 'I knew I forgot something. Cuff her, Constable.'

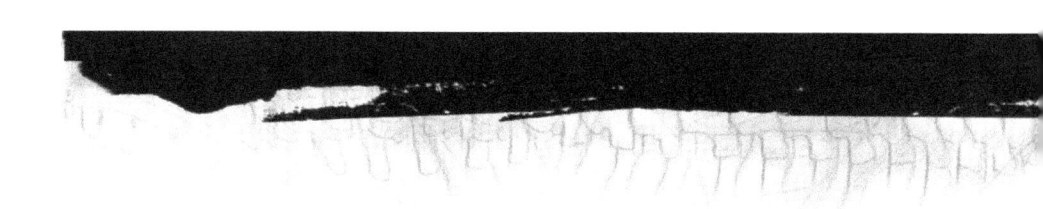

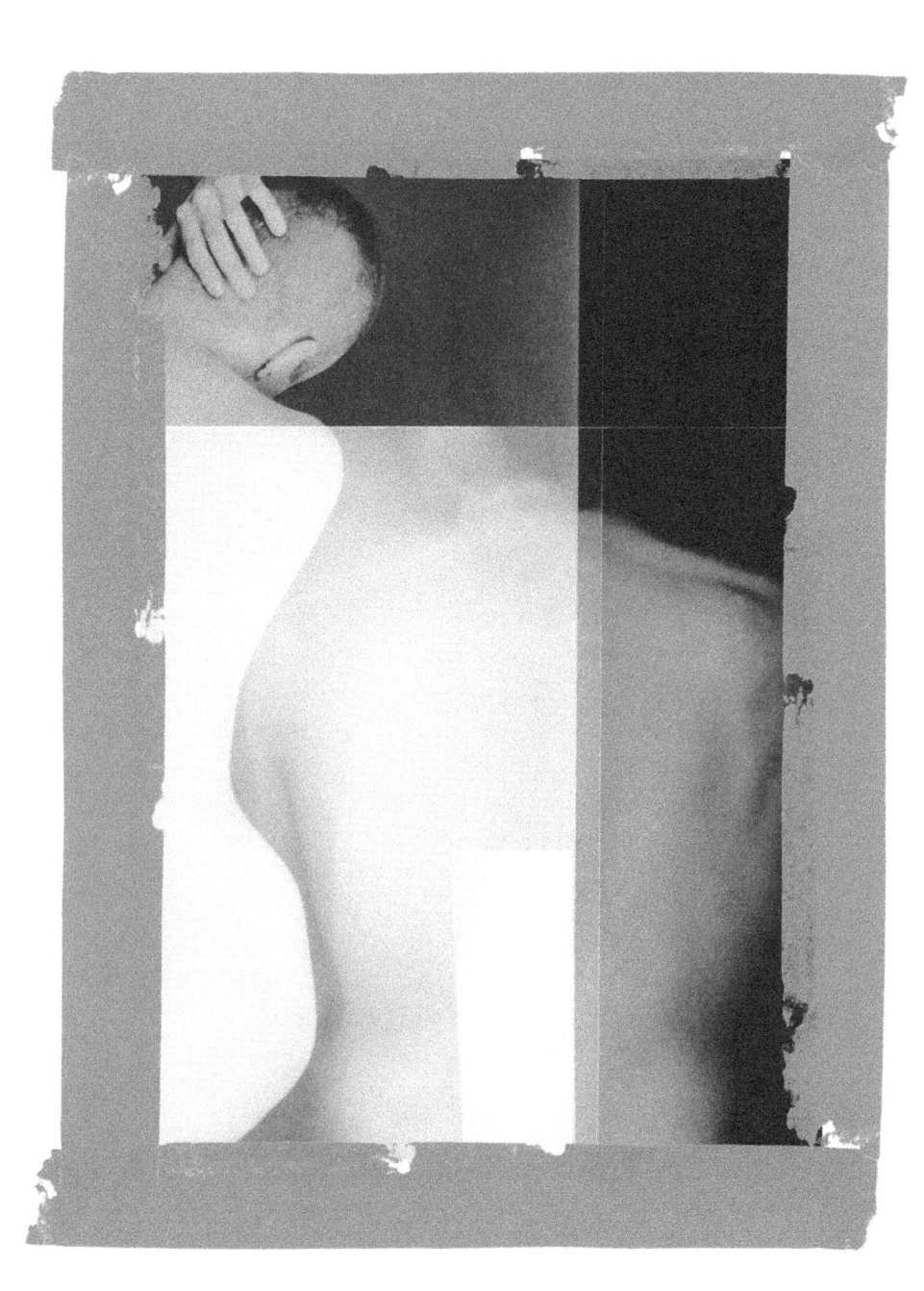

BLIND DATE

by Pam Corsie

James unhooked the heel of his brogues from the middle bar of the railings he was leaning against. He placed his right foot firmly on the ground and transferred his, not insubstantial, weight from his left leg and hooked the heel of his left brogue over the middle bar. Nonchalance did not come easily to James and trying to look unconcerned was proving difficult. He glanced at his watch and was amazed again at how slowly time moved when he was waiting for someone, yet raced by when he was enjoying himself.

I was only a couple of minutes late, he thought. Surely she could have waited a couple of minutes. It was now nine minutes since the rendezvous time. Perhaps she walked past me and thought I didn't look like her type, whatever he is. That was the trouble with blind dates, you never knew who was going to turn up. All that GSOH, OHAC, positive outlook on life, and a photograph that could be ten years out of date, or of somebody else, on dating sites was all very well, but it wasn't until you met someone face to face that you really knew who you were getting.

I'll give her until fifteen minutes have gone by and then I'm off, he thought. As his eyes darted left and right along the High Street, in his peripheral vision he noticed a very attractive young woman. She was sitting alone at a table for two outside the cafe. Mmm, he thought, watching her blonde hair wafting gently in the breeze, dark glasses, pretty red summer dress long enough to be discreet, short enough to be beguiling. As she uncrossed and re-crossed her slender legs he clocked matching red sandals. Her large handbag was flopped against the table leg and the shoulder strap rested in her hand in her lap.

Cautious type, he thought. No one's going to grab her bag from under the table in this part of town! He checked the time. Wow, that six minutes had just flown by as he was admiring the lady in red. And then it hit him. Red, she said she'd be wearing red. This vision of loveliness must be his blind date.

He stood up straight and squared his shoulders. He could hear Mum saying, 'Don't slouch James, it looks so uncouth.' Hoping desperately that she hadn't spotted him staring, he walked purposefully across the pavement towards her.

'Hi, I'm James,' he held out his hand. She turned to face him and bestowed a brilliant smile.

'Hello James, I'm Annabelle, nice to meet you.' She made no attempt to shake his proffered hand, which confused James for a minute. Then he realised she was probably waiting for the mwah, mwah kiss greeting so favoured by people who wore enormous sunglasses. Happily, he leaned forward and did the honours. Annabelle smiled again; it was going well.

'You smell nice,' she said. 'Present? Or do you have to buy your own aftershave?' I'd better not tell her Mum bought it for me for Christmas, he thought.

'May I join you?' he asked, pulling out a chair.

'I thought that was the idea,' she replied, her gorgeous lips curled upward at the corners of her mouth in another smile.

I am such a prat, thought James, useless at this dating game.

'I was beginning to think you weren't coming,' she said. She picked nervously at the hem of her red dress. 'I did wonder if you'd spotted me and kept walking, congratulating yourself on a lucky escape.'

'Lucky escape! I'm feeling really lucky just now. I'm sorry I was late. I didn't realise that meeting outside the cafe meant you'd be sitting at a table. I was leaning against the railings over there thinking I'd blown it, or you'd blown me out.'

Annabelle leaned back in her chair and laughed, a tinkly, uncritical chuckle that made James glad he had sat down as his legs turned to jelly. 'What would you like to drink?' he asked, hoping his legs would get him safely to the cafe's counter.

'A hot chocolate. Even though it's sunny, I love whipped cream and marshmallows,' she replied, licking her lips.

James walked fairly steadily to the counter thinking, thank heavens she didn't order a decaf skinny latte or one of those other excuses for a drink. Hot chocolate, whipped cream and marshmallows, she's a girl after my own heart. Although he had to admit she didn't look as though she had drunk quite as many as he had.

He placed the hot chocolate with all the trimmings in front of Annabelle on the table and, by the time he had settled on the chair next to her, she was already tucking in and had a whipped cream moustache. He laughed gently and leaned across to wipe the cream away. She jumped as he caressed her top lip. 'Sorry,' he said, 'but you've got cream on your top lip. I was just trying to help.'

'I'm sorry too James, I didn't mean to appear rude. I was just not ready for that.'

Slow down James, don't presume, take it steady, he remonstrated with himself.

After another hot chocolate each that Annabelle insisted on paying for, but James insisted on collecting from the counter, she said she'd had a lovely morning but was meeting her mother for lunch so she really ought to leave. During the speediest morning of James's life their conversation had rapidly progressed to funny anecdotes about their over-protective parents. James understood that Annabelle could not cancel lunch with her mother who needed to confirm that James had turned up to meet her daughter and then behaved himself.

'Can I see you again?' he asked a little nervously. 'We seem to be getting on very well, I've really enjoyed this morning.'

'Well, if you're sure you want to, James. I can be a bit of a liability sometimes.'

'I find that hard to believe. You've been perfect company this morning. You even paid for two of the hot chocolates, I call that an asset not a liability,' he laughed.

'In that case, how about Sunday lunch, tomorrow? The Coach and Horses at one?'

'Sounds good to me,' grinned James.

'Don't be late James, and I'll bring my purse,' she laughed and patted his thigh where it rested against hers.

As they stood, Annabelle lifted her cavernous bag from the floor and pulled out a short stick. With a flick of her wrist, like a magic wand, the stick sprung outwards and formed a full-size white pole that she moved from side to side in front of her. 'Shall I hail you a cab?' James asked.

'That would be lovely, thank you.'

The cab pulled up next to a gap in the railings, James kissed Annabelle on her cheek and handed her into the back seat. 'Have a good lunch. Make sure you tell your mum about my good points. See you tomorrow, I'm looking forward to it already.'

'Me too,' said Annabelle.

Best blind date ever, thought James as he strolled along the High Street, a spring in his step. He glanced at his reflection in a shop window, squared his shoulders and pulled in his stomach. If he could have done an Eric Morecambe jump and heel-click step he would have.

***

'Hello darling,' called Joyce as her daughter entered the bar. She strolled across the room, her heels clicking and clacking on the hard surface. Annabelle must have heard her coming above the general hubbub in the busy pub, as she turned and started to make her way towards her mother, leaving the sanctuary of the porch where the taxi driver had left her. 'You've been gone a while, so I guess he turned up?' Joyce said warily.

'Yes, Mum, he turned up. I've had a really good morning.'

'I'm pleased to hear it, Belle. It was about time someone half decent came from that dating agency. All that money and they've been nothing but dead beats so far.'

'Oh, Mum! They weren't all dead beats. In fact, some of them were rather nice.'

'That's as may be, but not one of them hung around long enough to get past your, y'know, er... um...'

'Inability to see very much? I think that's the expression you're fumbling for. I know I'm virtually blind, Mum, why you can't just say it I don't know. It's not as though I've done something disgraceful. Perhaps if my accident had resulted in a missing limb or facial disfigurement you would have been happier.'

Annabelle and Joyce had this conversation regularly. Annabelle knew her mum found it difficult to look at her beautiful daughter without being confused that the first impression of a perfect, healthy young woman completely masked her inability to see. Joyce felt that if Annabelle's visual impairment was more obvious then potential suitors would know what they were dealing with straightaway and Belle would not suffer the awkwardness of having to explain and then endure the pain of waiting in vain for that phone call or text asking for a second date. But Annabelle insisted on first dates being on as equal a footing as she could orchestrate. The last thing she needed was pity. She wanted a man to look at her and think, she is gorgeous, not she is blind.

'Actually Mum, I didn't mention it and neither did James. The time just flew by. We laughed a lot and were so comfortable with each other that I just stood up and got my cane out of my bag, as though we were old friends, and he already knew everything about me.'

'Didn't he say anything?'

'Like what? Oh crumbs, you're blind! What would be the point of that, I already know I can't see.'

'Don't be a smart-mouth, Annabelle. I worry about you. If and when you're a mum you'll worry about your children, it's what mums are for and what they do well.'

'I'm sorry, Mum. I know you worry about me, but there is no need, not with James anyway. He was a natural. He just took my arm, flagged a cab and put me in it. And, we've already arranged to have lunch tomorrow, so no waiting, clutching my mobile and chewing my nails.'

'Where are you having lunch, Belle? Not too far away, I hope. Sundays are busy for us, it may be difficult to get away to drop you off.'

'No worries, Mum. The Coach and Horses does the best Sunday lunch in town. I can have extra roasties cooked by dad and the familiarity of my own home. I may have failed to mention to James that the Coach was our pub, but I thought you'd like to meet him. I thought you could tell me what he looks like. I might not be able to see him myself but I do have standards, you know.'

Joyce leaned back in her chair and laughed. Why did she worry about Annabelle? She was the most positive person Joyce knew and despite only having 15% vision, had never lost her self-confidence for long, even during the awful time immediately after her accident.

As the waitress walked across the bar with their regular order, she found herself looking forward to meeting James. Given the way he dealt with the white stick he was either the epitome of cool, or as blind as a bat himself.

***

'Hi Mum, I'm home,' called James.

'Did you have a good time? What was she like? She did turn up, didn't she?' Ellen asked.

'Of course she turned up, who could resist a blind date with me?'

'Well, I could. That profile on the web-site didn't exactly make you sound exciting and your aunty Janet told me she thought the photograph you uploaded was a bit scruffy.'

'Love me, love my every slovenly mannerism.' He skipped up behind Ellen, put his arms round her waist and picked her up.

'Aaah, hey, put me down you big soft lump. What's going on? You're behaving like you've won the lottery.'

'This must be just how it feels,' gushed James. 'I'm so happy. She was gorgeous – long blonde hair, slim, beautiful smile, well dressed. What more could a handsome young man like me ask for?'

'Does she have a name?'

'Annabelle, classy, it suits her perfectly.'

'Glass of wine with lunch to celebrate perhaps?'

'Good idea. Is there a bottle in the fridge?'

'There is, I had a good feeling about this one, so I put a bottle in when you left for your date, just in case you wanted to celebrate.' Ellen didn't mention to James that this bottle had been in and out of the fridge like a yo-yo since he joined the dating agency. Some things mums liked to keep to themselves!

'Lunch will be a few minutes,' James said. 'Have you fed Honey?'

'Fed, watered and ready to go. I'm meeting Aunty Janet so I want all the goss, as Janet's sure to ask.'

'We're having salad. On the way home I spotted my reflection in a shop window. I should make more of an effort, stand up straight, get a bit fitter, maybe lose a few pounds. Annabelle deserves to be seen with someone in better shape than me, even though she'd struggle to meet anyone else with such a heady mixture of scintillating personality and intoxicating good looks!'

Ellen laughed. He really was incorrigible and funny and sweet and kind and she hoped this Annabelle wasn't going to lead him on and then break his heart. Mums and their sons, she thought. Were mums and their daughters on a more equal footing?

'And, we're having lunch tomorrow. 1pm at the Coach and Horses. I don't think I'll be having salad though, the chef's roasties are legendary.'

***

'Annabelle, stop mooning about, come here and dry some glasses for us please, darling.'

'He'd better turn up,' Joyce said to one of the regulars. 'I'll have his guts for garters if he hurts my girl.'

The regular smiled, he'd seen Joyce turn out many a drunk on a Saturday night. He didn't give much for the lad's chances if he messed around with the lovely Annabelle.

Joyce blow dried Annabelle's blonde hair and left it curling loosely about her shoulders. She carefully applied a thin layer of foundation to Belle's flawless skin, a little mascara and brushed on the red lipstick.

'Don't want to gild the lily,' she said quietly.

Annabelle smiled, 'You always say that, Mum.'

'Well, beauty needs no adornment.'

Another favourite, thought Annabelle. She blew a kiss in her mother's direction. What would she do without her and dad? She was glad she had suggested having lunch at the Coach and Horses.

Meanwhile, James stepped out of the shower, liberally splashing himself with after shave.

As he tucked his pale blue buttoned-collar shirt into the waistband of his chinos, he turned sideways in front of the mirror and sucked in his tummy. 'Grrrr,' he growled. 'Go get her, tiger.'

'Crikey James, if that's the best chat-up line you can manage you'd better stay home.'

'What are you doing in my room?'

'What are you up to? I can always tell when you are keeping something from me.'

'Nothing for you to worry about, old girl,' he said and he pinched her cheeks as he went past her. 'I'll give you the complete heads up when I get back.'

James entered the Coach and Horses, strolled to the bar and asked for a table for two. The barmaid came from behind the bar to take him to the table, and, as if by magic, a smiling Annabelle appeared at her side. 'Hello Annabelle,' brayed James. Oh crumbs, a bit enthusiastic, James cringed inwardly.

'Hello James,' replied Annabelle, rather more restrained, but he could tell from her smile she was delighted he'd come. He took her arm and they followed Joyce to the table in the window. 'Thank you,' said Annabelle to the barmaid.

'You're welcome Bel–.... er Miss.'

'I think she knew you. Do you come here often?'

'Ha ha ha, that is such a lame chat-up line,' laughed Annabelle. 'I bet you say that to all the girls.'

'Well, it was better than the line I practised at home,' answered James. 'I hear the Sunday lunch is delicious and the roasties second to none. Shall we go for the carvery?'

'I'm not great at helping myself to food. I may need some assistance to make sure all my vegetables make it safely onto the plate and the gravy doesn't end up on my shoes.'

'Not a problem,' breezed James. 'I waited at tables for extra cash when I was at uni. Two plates piled with roast meat, vegetables and gravy will be a breeze. You may even feel the need to leave a tip!'

They ordered with the waitress, James poured them each a glass of wine and put the bottle back in the cooler. 'Cheers.' Annabelle lifted her glass and held it steady whilst James clinked his against it.

'Cheers to you too, beautiful lady.'

The chef behind the carvery nodded to let James know that he was ready when they were. With mock gallantry James held Annabelle's chair as she stood and he took her elbow. They both chose roast beef and James loaded their plates with vegetables.

Lunch was delicious. The beef was succulent and, as James checked Annabelle's plate to make sure she was enjoying it too, he noticed that her beef was already cut into bite-sized pieces and she was relishing the mouth-watering meal.

'Generous portions,' mumbled James. 'Wonderful roasties. We'll have to come here again.'

Again, thought Annabelle. He wants to see me again! 'I'm sure we will,' she muttered coyly.

As he put his cutlery together on his empty plate, James looked at the chef, still on duty behind the carvery, and gave him a thumbs up. The chef smiled and winked. The barmaid was standing very close to the chef and grinning like a Cheshire cat.

'I think the chef and the waitress are more than colleagues, Annabelle!'

'I hope so,' laughed Annabelle, 'they're my parents. This is my family's pub!'

'What, you've got me here under false pretences in order to meet your parents?' She wants me to meet her mum and dad, he thought gleefully. 'Perhaps you'd better invite them over, would they join us for pud or coffee? I was going to try and give up the sweet things, but that would mean you too, and I couldn't possibly do that.'

Annabelle rolled her eyes at another of his corny chat-up lines and laughed.

'James,' said George, as he extended his hand, 'a pleasure to meet you.'

'And you too, sir,' responded James, giving George's hand a firm shake.

'My husband is George and I'm Joyce,' said Annabelle's mum.

'Delighted,' said James as he leant forward and gave Joyce the mwah mwah kiss greeting that he knew the women in this family preferred. I'm really getting the hang of this, he thought smugly. 'Would you care to join us?'

George and Joyce each grabbed a chair from nearby tables. A waitress appeared with a tray of four dessert plates each holding a different pudding. 'House specialities,' said George. 'Puds to share, dig in.'

After the creamy, crunchy and chocolatey puddings disappeared George and Joyce went back to work. 'He seems okay,' said George. 'He seems to instinctively know how to get the best out of our Belle. Are you sure he hasn't spoken to her about her sight?'

'Well, up until he arrived for lunch I know he hadn't mentioned it to Belle. Did you notice how he placed her plate directly in front of her and gently rested her hand over the spoon so she didn't have to search for it? The way he topped up her wine glass and then put it back in exactly the same place was so thoughtful. And he was soooo handsome, Belle will be chuffed when I tell her.'

'Not exactly slim though, was he?'

'You're a fine one to talk, George,' laughed Joyce, affectionately patting her husband on his publican's belly.

'Mum and Dad like you, James.'

'How can you tell? They were very polite, but then so was I, it's difficult to work out what anyone is thinking when they're being polite.'

'They would still be sat here, guarding me, grim-faced and silently challenging you to stay, if they hadn't liked you.'

'You, my sweet Belle, I liked it when they called you that, are going to have to run the gauntlet with my mother soon.'

'Shall we go for a walk in the sunshine, James? It's a beautiful afternoon.'

'Good idea, and we could make plans for another date. How long do you think you can wait before you see me again?'

The hall clock was striking five as James let himself into the bungalow he shared with his mum. He walked into the sitting room and crossed to the window where Ellen was enjoying the last of the afternoon's sun. 'Delicious lunch,' said James, rubbing his hands across his tummy. 'I could be tempted back there.'

'Just for the food, or maybe for Annabelle? Come on, I'm all ears and Aunty Janet will be waiting by the phone for an update.'

'Well,' said James, relaxing back into his chair, 'you can tell Aunty Janet that I had a very successful second date. So successful was our first date, that on the second, Annabelle arranged for me to meet her parents.'

'What?! She's keen.'

'It's not quite as it sounds. The Coach and Horses is her family's pub. They worry about her, so she thought she'd fix it so they could see me in action and put their minds at rest, that I was not some sort of mad axe murderer.'

'Your stomach must have flipped when she told you what she had planned.'

'Actually, it worked rather well as she didn't let on until after we had finished our mains. By then, of course, we were quite relaxed and they joined us for puds and coffee. I didn't really have time to panic.

'I thought perhaps she could come to dinner on Wednesday evening. I'll meet her after work and bring her round. Are you okay with that, Mum?'

'Fine by me,' replied Ellen. She really wanted to throw a hat in the air, whoop with glee and dance a jig. James was finally bringing home a girl to meet her.

***

Ellen heard James unlock the front door, 'Welcome to our home. Come and meet my mum.'

James led Annabelle into the sitting room. Every step found her preparing for a handshake or a hug from James's mum. None was forthcoming. Perhaps she's not so keen on meeting me after all, thought Belle. But a cheery voice called, 'Hello my dear, come in, come in. I'm Ellen.' James guided Annabelle across the uncluttered room to the chair at the window opposite his mum. Gently he placed her right hand in Ellen's right hand. 'Mum, meet Annabelle, Belle, meet Ellen,' he said quietly. Honey stretched, stood slowly and sniffed Annabelle thoroughly.

'Don't take any notice of Honey, dear,' said Ellen, 'she's just checking you out. I hope you like dogs. Honey is a working dog, she's my eyes since I lost my sight. I'd be stuck without her.'

No wonder he was so good with me, thought Annabelle, and said, 'I can't see either, or rather I have 15% vision. James didn't tell me you couldn't see, Ellen.'

'And he didn't tell me about your poor sight either,' said Ellen. 'But then it's not the most important thing about either of us, is it?'

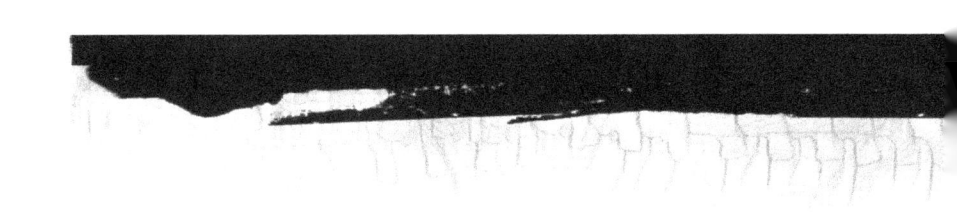

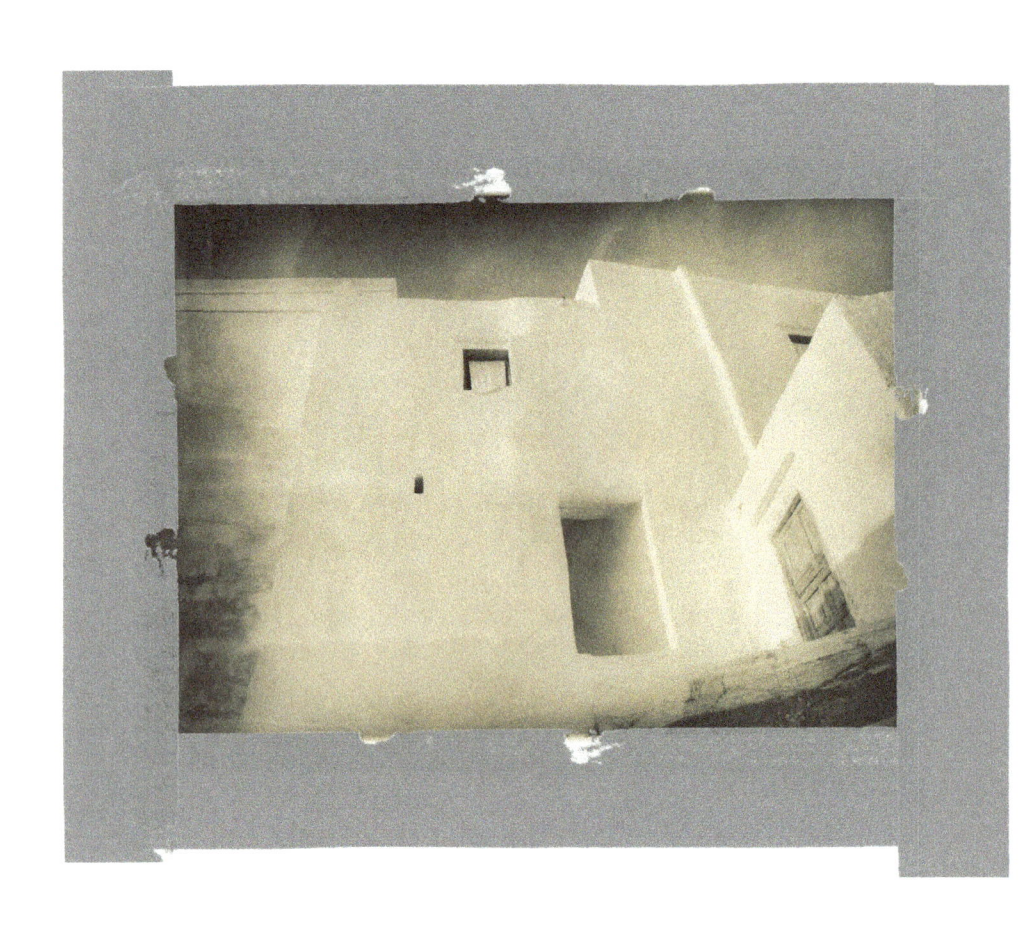

COLD CALLING

by Claire Goodman

Bad back, grey hair, stiff hands. I try to straighten up. Crack crack. Cup of tea, yesterday's paper. Quick sit down. Sip of tea.
 Too hot. Said Eileen.
 I look at the clock, 10am and no breakfast. Just getting started and to-do list as long as my arm.
 You should make a start? She suggested.
 I nod and force a smile. Gas bill, gas bill. Must go today. The lettering gone from black to red. I pause and look at the front door on my way through the hall. Front door, gas bill. To-bloody-day.
 You haven't even had breakfast, she says. Gentle scolding. It's okay for her. Always fine, hair set, permanently ready.
 I nod thanks in her direction, wave an arm over the singed toast.
 I wonder can I eat –
 You need to change the setting. She gently scolds. She moves to the toaster. Always right, always in charge.

I'm at the window. I hear voices. Panic. Hold my breath, frozen. Hold it in. Breathe out, drop tea bag. I rest my head on the cupboard, allow myself a moment of despair.
 Eileen is about to say something, some kind words of encouragement.

Doorbell rings. I jump, ask the wife, are we expecting anyone? We are not expecting anyone. Kitchen doorway, hello old friend. I've done this before. I peer into the hall. I look through the frosted glass either side of the door and make out the shape of a person. One person, two people. Two people chatting. The bell rings again, I wince. Ridiculous, silly old. Back hurts more.

They disappear, off down the garden path. At the kitchen window I see the two bodies, heads now cut off by the overgrown hedge.

I sigh. I lean. I turn round. Rub an old dry stiff hand. Burnt toast.

She stands at the bottom of the stairs. Eileen stands, patience. Years of patience, that one. I motivate myself. Bag, list, check this and that. Count to ten. Check again. I creak upstairs. Stand at the top to get my breath. Dry hand running through thin hair. Did I open the windows up here I wonder. Breathe.

None of the windows are open up here. She said. I know this. I will check anyway.

I make a deal with her. She smiles in agreement. Walk down the stairs, pick up the bag and list and open the front door. The quicker you do it the sooner it will be done.

I walk slowly, a deep exhale. Bag in hand, preoccupied. I open the front door.

'Have you heard the good news,' said the stranger in front of me. Sudden daylight. Neither myself or Eileen had heard it.

I'm greeted by a lady in a purple coat, shiny hair, good news and eager. She smiles, she is waiting for my reply. I don't have it. I look around her. Path in front of me, shops. Bills to pay. Black. Today. Red.

I make to retreat, steadying myself by the door. Face frozen. Stranger lady shifts the book. She is going to read the good news but I don't want to hear it. I edge into the house, looking down at the floor. I close the door, so softly it doesn't even click. I frown.

Soon I hear the creak of the gate and watch the purple shadow of her coat disappearing through the frosted glass.

Maybe try again later. Said my dead wife.

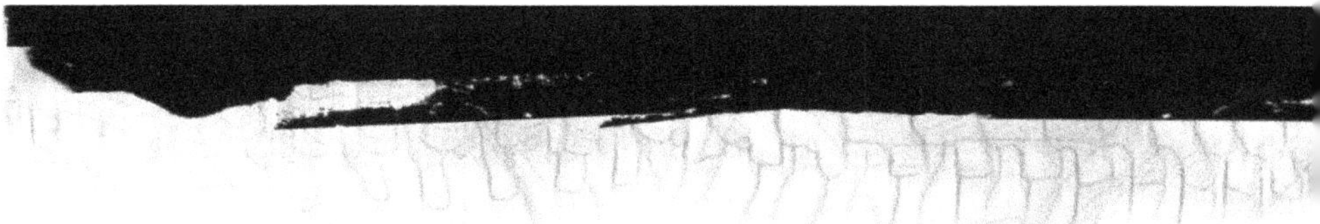

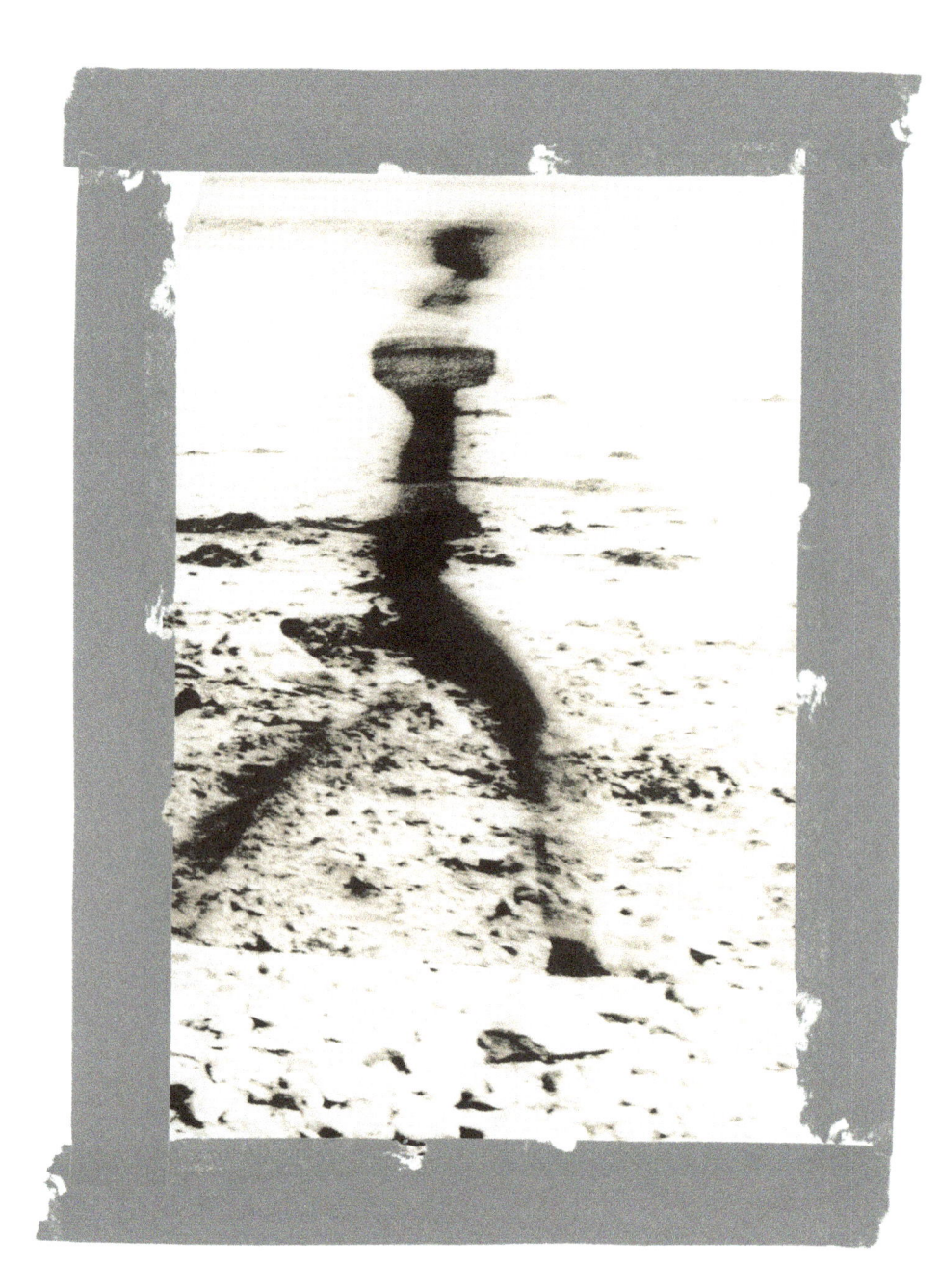

FARMER YOUNG

by Jamie Harding

Farmer Young had a medium-sized farm, on which his piggery was his pride and joy. He had owned his farm, he would tell people, for many, many years, but, he would add with a twinkle in his eye, the piggery only for many years. And over the course of these many years, Farmer Young's joy of his piggery meant that it became his first farming port of call each morning, once Ronald, his cockerel, had proudly announced the new day with his quite tremendous crowing.

Farmer Young would struggle to admit that he liked Ronald's impossibly loud alarm as it rebounded throughout the barns and outbuildings, but he would concede that it was very, very effective. And once Ronald's soundwaves had finally petered out, and the various human and animal heartbeats around the farm had returned to a normal rate, and Farmer Young had stirred the sleep from his eyes and bid his also-rising wife a sleepy good morning dearest, he could undertake his morning routine.

Rising together, Farmer Young and his wife took it in turns to draw the curtains each day, and allow the warmth of the sun, if there was any around, to spill into their bedroom. If it was very cold weather, they may have filled their bedroom's small fireplace with kindling and old newspaper from the basket on the hearth the previous evening, and left it to smoulder and glow and crackle itself out overnight. Old houses, especially old farmhouses, were designed with a certain warmth and robustness in mind, Farmer Young often mused, sparing a thought for those whose houses were reliant on distinctly impersonal central heating systems.

When the couple had risen and drawn, they would clad themselves in dressing gowns, and wander along the hallway to the bathroom to wash their faces and brush their teeth, side by side, in the twin, cream-coloured sinks that had stood in the farmhouse since it was built. Farmer Young's wife would then insist that he take his ration of pills that the doctor had prescribed, as he wasn't terribly good at remembering.

I don't want you to be like you were when they took the pigs that last time, Farmer Young's wife would often tell her husband, her hand gently laid on his arm, his weak smile braver than she knew.

With their teeth cleaned, their faces scrubbed and Farmer Young's pills gulped down, the couple would then carrying out all of their other necessary morning bathroom business – in Farmer Young's case, this was to be carried out in the little bathroom adjoined to the guest bedroom on his wife's grave insistence, who after several years of morning disharmony concerning the matter, refused to let him use the same bathroom as her for what she called his morning unpleasantness.

I love you, but I could never love what that bottom of yours is capable of, his wife had told him on many an occasion. But by having been sequestered to a little bathroom of his own for his morning unpleasantness, Farmer Young had shrewdly turned his ostracization into an indulgence for paperback novels. The little bathroom had become a miniature library of sorts, featuring as it did a very long and wobbly shelf chaotically lined with paperbacks that Farmer Young had picked up for 50p here or even £1 there, if it was a big one, from the surrounding towns' charity shops and jumble sales.

Pushing his way into the little bathroom each morning, Farmer Young would glance at his paperbacks, recognizing each of them with all their different spine colours and titles in a variety of fonts, author's names, and the pleasant memories of a good read that stirred within him upon casting his sleepy morning eyes along the haphazard row.

Farmer Young loved all different sorts of tales, and would happily dip into macabre collections of ghost stories, or perhaps become engrossed by any one of his number of coldly-written spy novels whose protagonists seemed to be forever wandering around desolate, rainy European cities and meeting austere men in hats. Once they met, they were always swapping information or money, or chasing or, occasionally, even killing a person, or helping to bring down an oppressive regime – all of this in between seducing impressionable young ladies, or coming up with imaginative ways to break into hotel rooms, or checking if their own hotel room had been imaginatively broken into.

So it was a variety of fiction that entertained Farmer Young as he carried out his morning duties in that little bathroom, and often he would be sat reading, lost in some tall tale or other, long after his movement had finished and his bottom had gotten very cold and pins and needles had started to make his legs feel all fuzzy, and his wife would be calling from the landing, breezily imploring Farmer Young to join her and the rest of the country in doing something constructive with his day.

At this, Farmer Young would quietly grumble, get to an appropriate part of the story, close the crinkly pages of his paperback after inserting his tattered old leather bookmark band and finish up in the little bathroom, already eagerly anticipating the next morning's ghostly tale, or love story, or high seas caper.

The books' pages, which were generally already old and yellowing, had been made yet more crinkled and brittle by the slightly damp conditions of the little bathroom, and each morning he would weakly pledge to take the books back to a charity shop so that its cycle of fundraising could continue, and furthermore, that he would pay a man from Barry's Electricals – maybe even Barry himself, should he be bothered – to install an extractor fan.

Farmer Young and his wife would then amble downstairs together, smiling upon hearing the faint padding of paws and clacking of claws as their ageing Jack Russell, Percy, and even more ageing Persian cat, Prunella, rose to either immediately prowl towards their food bowl (Prunella), or stiffly amble over to the Youngs, offering a cold, wet nose, a warm tongue, and a coyly waggling tail (Percy).

Farmer Young and his wife would oblige their pets with an affectionate dispensing of strokes and cooed greetings, before teaming up to pour fresh water for them both and fork morsels of expensive, juicy meat that Percy and Prunella's desirous, imploring faces had subconsciously persuaded Farmer Young into buying over at the animal feed shop near the station.

Once his regular weekday breakfast of thickly-buttered toast topped with a dollop of homemade raspberry or gooseberry jam had been washed down with a huge mug of strong, sweet tea, it was time for Farmer Young to pull on his wellington boots, whistle Percy to his paws, and open the very old, very creaky front door and set off to the piggery to begin his daily chores. His wife would wish him a nice day's work as her husband and Percy sauntered away. As she sploshed hot, foaming water over the breakfast crockery, 60's and 70's easy listening classics drifted from the wireless.

Now undoubtedly the head pet of the house, Prunella would slink across the kitchen's large flagstone tiles, mulling over whether to snootily inspect Percy's bowl for leftover snippets of meat that she could somewhat less-than-snootily nibble at, or simply to laze about on a comfortable-looking sofa or an inviting, freshly-made bed until entertainment presented itself to her.

A busy weekday was a fine thing for Farmer Young – seeing to the needs of his animals, before returning to the farmhouse for one of his wife's hot, cooked dinners, after which he would go over his farming administration whilst sipping on a huge, steaming mug of coffee. However, they didn't compare to his weekends, and especially his Saturdays. 'Almost the king of the days, dearest,' Farmer Young would declare to his wife as early in the week as Wednesday afternoon, as he looked ahead to his weekend.

Farmer Young truly loved Saturdays. The week would always have been busy, and the weekends not too different – but, come Saturday, he allowed himself an extra thirty minutes snoozing in bed once Ronald had crowed. Then, Farmer Young would snuggle up with his wife, whilst the weather shone, rained, or blew outside. Farmer Young loved to slip off his pyjamas, gently raise his wife's nightie, and nestle his thighs against her milky, round, bottom cheeks before whispering sweet words into her ear, his huge, shovel-like hands beginning to slowly explore her curves. 'Oh James,' she would softly reply, in an amenable voice. Some Saturdays, anyhow.

Saturday breakfasts were another boon of the weekend's arrival. After their extra minutes in bed, and the increased rush of endorphins that were sizzling between Farmer Young and his wife, a full and scrumptious breakfast was called for. Enormous speckled eggs, freshly fetched from his team of free-range hens were cracked open by his wife and poured onto a sizzling pool of butter in the almighty frying pan. These, huge, pure white splats of egg were soon slipping around the pan, crowned by large, deep, orange yolks that somehow managed not to burst and ooze out until Farmer Young poked them with his fork. Then they were ready to be joined on Farmer Young's breakfast plate by a brace of thick, grilled sausages and halves of tomato, a large scoop of baked beans, and whatever else his wife had managed to concoct.

But the king of days would still involve a heavy dose of farming, and after letting his breakfast sink down, whilst perusing the local paper and discussing the day ahead with his wife, Farmer Young, ably assisted by Percy, now had work to do, and the piggery was calling.

Farmer Young had played around with his piggery routine over the years, but it invariably started with him striding inside the cavernous pig-house and roaring a 'Good morning, my perky porkers!' to his excitable pigs, before inspecting each pen for signs of overnight trouble and reaching inside to give each and every pig – except for the shy ones – a tickle or pat if he could reach. For their part, the pigs responded by snuffling Farmer Young's oversized fingers, oinking – or in some cases, eerily screeching – their souls out in anticipation of eating their swill or 'Tottenham pudding 2.0', as Farmer Young futuristically insisted on calling the swirled mishmash mixed with modern pig feed that comprised their breakfast. Whilst they had never managed to raise little beings of their own, Farmer Young and his wife had always looked upon their animals as their family, however hard it was at times to raise them, and to let go.

For the warmer months, Farmer Young had knocked up two dozen or so pig-houses for his three dozen or so pigs out of corrugated iron and lengths of spare timber. The pigs were free to roam a two-acre field, filled with water troughs, rudimentary scratching posts (he'd once noticed a friendly little piglet that he'd let into the farmhouse having a grand time itching away on Prunella's post, much to his wife's and the cat's chagrin), made from old, rounded fenceposts. Farmer Young would painstakingly check for splintering to ensure that the scratching didn't lead to any nasty scrapes, and scatter piles of straw and hay about for the pigs to dry themselves once they'd finished rolling in the huge mud-puddles that were nature's contribution to the pigs' fairweather lodgings.

The passing motorists enjoyed gazing at the young animals' frolicking, and always laughed, or at least smiled upon reading a large sign in the field that Farmer Young had erected after a moderate brainwave early one spring: New Pork City, it said.

The farmer/animal relationship was always sunny the day New Pork City re-welcomed its seasonal citizens, and remained pleasant until the City's middle noun and its financial implications meant that the field was missing both its happy pigs and Farmer Young's contented chuckling.

But, with it being deep into a particularly blowy, snowy and chilly winter season in which we now

catch up with Farmer Young, the pigs have been brought back in from their field to the piggery.

The pigs snuffle about in the snow, whilst he keeps a watchful eye on the strange, boisterous creatures with whom he shares

the farmland.

Farmer Young is attempting to reshuffle a few groups of pigs about, in

order to split up a couple of boys who seem to have taken something of an ear-nibbling dislike to each other overnight.

This performance has played out on countless mornings at the piggery, and today's extra

snap of cold
in the air has Farmer Young daydreaming of the forthcoming spring, and his pigs in their field,
and his bottom lip wobbles, and his heart flushes, as he momentarily recalls the horrible   fallout
that swarmed him the last time that
 they took the pigs.
He takes a moment to set himself,
and leans
against the piggery's feed room   door.
The crushing days which any farmer sees the animals he has reared, tended, cared
for
and fed are always bereft of chuckles, tickles and joy,
when they are collected and driven
away to the horrible place.
But these are farming facts of life Farmer Young thinks to himself, rather
fatalistically.
Images and memories of his time with the pigs run through Farmer Young's
mind, along with a few reassuring soundbites that he isn't sure if

he'd ever really believed in.
Well, I'm pleased to have known them and made their little houses and found toys for them. Shared   apples with
them. Varied their Tottenham pudding... And there will be more pigs, soon. More little souls, in pink, white, black and each with their own
 distinctive pigginess.

All will be okay.

These thoughts have been comforting Farmer Young for quite a few years now, although he
isn't really sure what comfort is meant to mean anymore.

Well then, Farmer Young had thought the last time he had surveyed the emptying fields, comfort me a-bloody-gain then. His huge hands had been restless, his fingers knitting themselves around each other, deep in the pockets of his itchy, baggy, not-very-comfortable-at-all-really trousers as he'd gazed at the disappearing, wiggly tails of his pigs, who were wondering just what on earth was going on. An impatient gaggle of men had unceremoniously hurried them onto the ramp of an ancient, grimy, double-decker lorry to be driven away to the horrible place, as black rain began to sweep through Farmer Young's mind.

And it had fallen long after the tailgate had been slammed shut, and the squeals of the pigs had grown fainter and fainter as the lorry had sped up the long track, spilling straw as it'd picked up speed, then slowed to turn onto the motorway, where it'd again sped along parallel with the empty New Pork City, until it disappearing from Farmer Young's view, and from his life.

Although the black rain was a regular caller to Farmer Young, that last time it had stretched on and on, until his wife had finally persuaded him to drive over to the town and consult with kindly old Dr Prentice, who had listened patiently to the couple describe how the twinkle had dulled in his eyes, and how his chuckle hadn't risen from his chest since they didn't know when. Leaving the surgery, Farmer Young had clutched his wife and a prescription for antidepressant medicines, which they'd then picked up from the town chemist to begin Farmer Young's recovery process.

Over the next few weeks, Farmer Young's tummy and brain and outlook on life had gotten used to the little white tablets as they'd fizzed through his system and aided his wife in restoring purpose and dignity to his work and his zeal.

I
thought I was   over allthis
silliness, thinksFarmerYoung astheblackrain   rages, and the coldnessof
the winter   wind   bites   at   his
     ageing

figure, and the fire in his eyes
dwindles.
Farmer Young now
moves from the feedroomdoor, and slumps down
against the first pen along.
A pair of particularlyinquisitive   floppyearedmale piglets
Immediately   bumble   overto
sniffleandsnuffle atthe peculiar   sight ofFarmer Young
down at their level. They nibble his
chequered farmer's shirt, and their increasingly
 frantic snuffling   with   their
snouts   lendshis
exposed forearms a smidgen of moist warmth,

b e f or e he eventually finds
 an empty pen,
and laysprone on a mixed bedofst raw, pig droppings, until he is joined at his side by a
confused and whimpering
Percy.
And there the pair lay,
surrounded   by a blanket of o   i   n
k   s,
and dabs of snow
that are blown in by
the biting winter wind.
When he has not turned up for a ladle or two of his favourite Saturday winter lunch – a simmering bowlful of thick vegetable soup accompanied by a doorstop-sized slice of heavily-buttered bread – Farmer Young's wife makes a rare foray into the depths of the farm, until, alerted by a cacophony of particularly excited oinking, she makes her way into the piggery.

Seeing Farmer Young and Percy flat out and shivering in the pen, her face drops, and she knows that the rain is falling again through her husband's mind.

Dropping to the floor, ignoring the droppings, Farmer Young's wife joins the pair, slides her arms around them as best she can, and waits for her husband to speak.

It's back, dearest. Those pills, I thought they worked, I thought I was back.

She tightens the huddle.

And now look where I've ended up. A silly old farmer, laid up in a bloody pig pen.... crying in the pig shit,

because I can't even.... I can't even BE a blummin' farmer.

She allows his words to breathe, and increasing her grip on her husband tighter yet, lets him feel her love.

You haven't ended up, James. You end up dead, we all end up dead, but you are living and flourishing now, and doing your best to make the circle of life that we've chosen to be as fair and as happy for these little beings as you can. You aren't owed anything except the chance to be the best that you can be, and boy oh boy I know how good, and loving and caring you are. I know it, James. I know.

He opens his eyes, and it seems that a

twinkling of love has been relit.

They clamber to their feet and paws, shoo the pigs back into their pens, and then go back to the farmhouse kitchen for a fine lunch of vegetable soup and bread.

Come the new spring, New Pork City's sign is taken down and burnt, along with some other bits and pieces that have been lying around on the farm not doing very much at all for far

too many years.

But the pigs are there, all three dozen of them. Farmer Young and his wife, Belinda's, three dozen pet pigs.

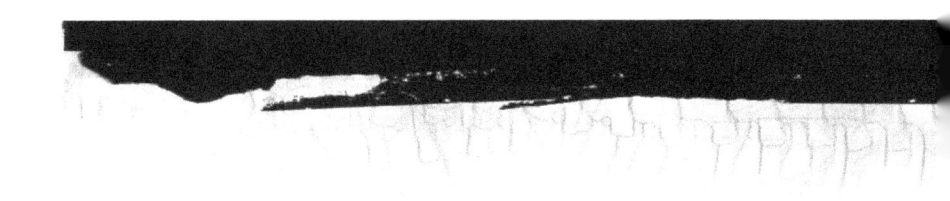

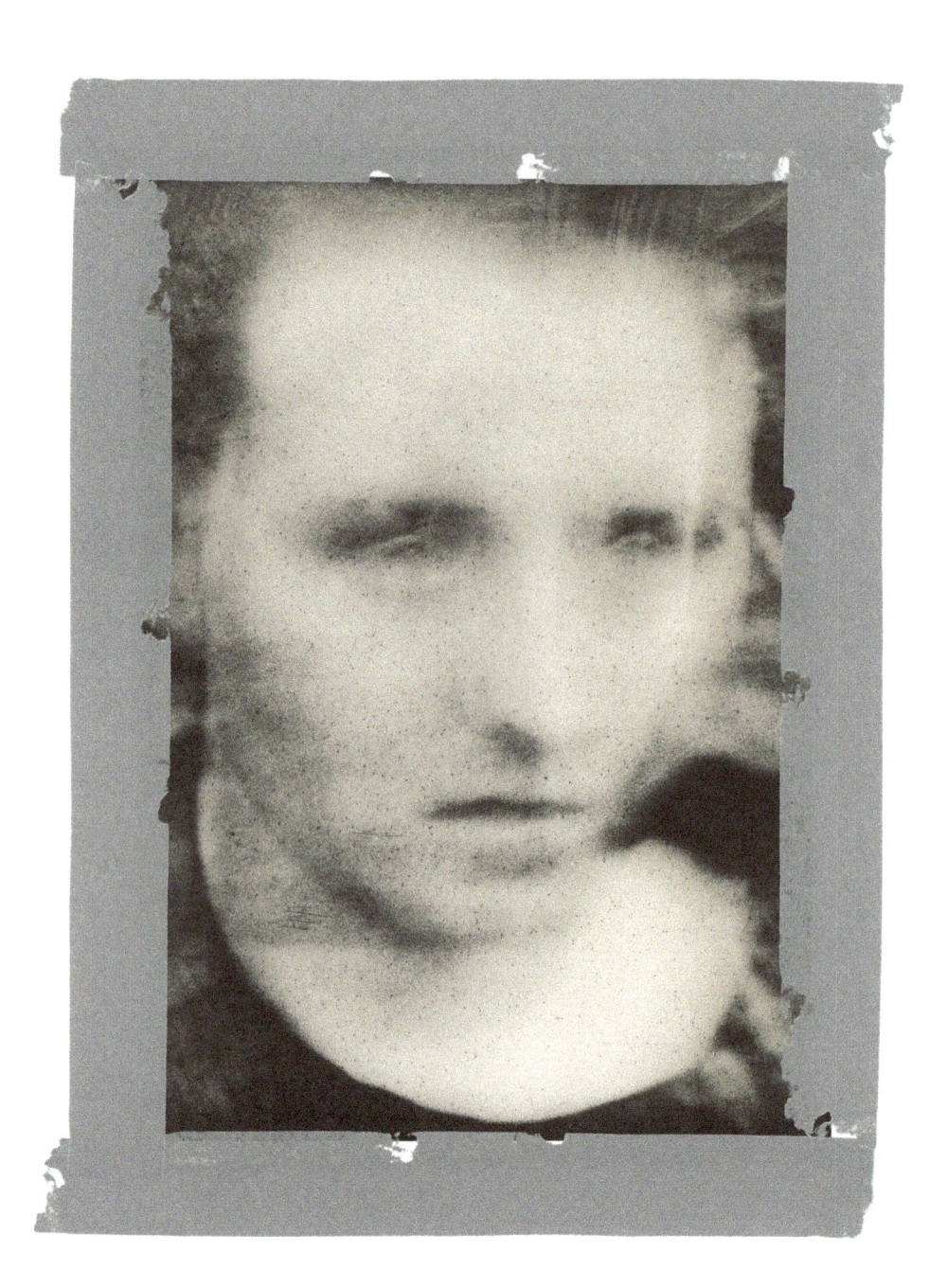

FOR STEVE

by Jim Knight

We stand in Times Square with the light from huge advertisement boards shifting across eyes that are wide like cartoon characters and unblinking. From street level you feel like you're a part of something and from up high you feel apart from everything. Those in penthouses look down from wrap-arounds and reflect on the insectile nature of all of us, finding fascination in the condos that are all beige and chrome. Where workers sit in shirts, shorts and socks in front of a TV that is never off and they sink in front of. Sometimes the workers will stand and look down too, after their eyes have been seeking high for too long and finding nothing. They reflect on us from less distance but in the same light. We stand and look up to them, feeling there is no one to look down on, but there is always subterranean. Steam pumps from huge vents and firemen sit atop their trucks breaking balls. Cool cops walk stooped on their beat smoking and winking, we remind ourselves that they're probably no different than the Met. Bueno, our cabbie, could be any working-class immigrant anywhere, but somehow he is only a New York cabbie, and he tells us he is middle-class because he has a car and a house and he doesn't have to use Medicaid – he has insurance. Bueno takes us into town over one of the famous bridges and through Queens. We ask him to take us down Wall Street and the mood is sombre. Where are the horns being sounded? Where are the monocles and top hats and flurries of money from cabs and the sloshing of scotch? It couldn't be seen anymore. It's like all of the fun was taken out of capitalism. It's all clinical now, surgical; young men in square specs and pressed suits with trust funds and allergies. I'd like to kill them all. The trash is not collected and the bar is open. We drink beer and eat red meat, we get the metro once and the stink and the soot is moreish. We were supposed to go one stop but we go three and back again to listen to the bullshit and weary after-work voices. New Yorkers, know your rights. If a loved one is detained or missing due to immigration problems, call the hotline. Three girls speak Spanish and one has a tongue piercing. She says, el niño, and points. There's a guy who sits alone at the side and throws black packages out of the doors to Hispanic youths who shove them in their pants and hop barriers, looking behind them. He doesn't look like much and I reckon if I had to, I could take him. The metro is really something. I'd liked to have cored out the tunnels with those blokes and be the first to ride it and get that first whiff of cologne and cigarette smoke – to stand shoulder to shoulder and know that the hoarse rumble through the tunnels would be owed only to us. We'd be proud. We sleep a little and the next morning we pick up a car from the other side of the park and soon we've left Manhattan. Yellow cabs and saloons dilute to flat beds and jeeps with sides sprayed in red mud. We stop at a town called Roscoe where the sign for a gun store jingles and Trump's face is everywhere. We open the door and the owner is called Lou, he has a T-shirt with an American bulldog on it and a 38-pistol strapped to his hip. Tattooed on his neck are two bullets, the tips of his fingers are yellowed and he blinks and laughs at us. You should see how my dad talks, he rocks on his toes and heels with his hands outstretched and fires out words. He won't stop until you've made a deal or had a fight or you're best friends. He and Lou are best friends, and they make a deal, they exchange caps and Lou says he's coming to the UK to take it back off him. The roads here are long and dip and curve past wooden homes and blackened barns. Some people must work here but no one does says Clay, the barkeep, who stands as every jaunty barkeep should, with the

FOR STEVE

NFL lighting him from behind, a towel over his shoulder and one hand on a clean bar he does not stop rubbing. We drive through the snowstorm with our heads down over the dash and our hands on top of the wheel, eyes looking straight into the throat of the beast like it's in the cab with us. We cross rivers and fords as quick as we dare and pass trucks overturned and snowed in, off the road. A driver stands outside drinking coffee from a trooper's flask, smoking cigarettes, his face is pink from the harshness of the wind and his lips are chapped because he licks them. We cruise past slow, voyeurs to his infortune but he doesn't seem to mind, pinching the base of his fur hood against the weather and turning, flicking the cigarette and climbing into the cab. The storm withdraws and the clouds are streaked like veins through ore and beyond them there is surely bluer sky and that's when the world opens up for us. You're driving right into the heart of something that's bigger than the storm but just as wild and dangerous and enticing. Ruddy Saxon faces trudge to cars and pumps and doors, their hands waving and their breath pluming. They're going to work or to school, or just to the drugstore to get a few things because it comes in thick and fast out here and you might not get another opportunity again. The storm is not the only beast out here. We watched a British bulldog kill three coyotes. He was chained to a stake and the coyotes were sniffing around his yard, they cornered a little dog, his companion. Their necks were raised up and bristling, trembling under a moon pale and clear. They advanced snarling. The little dog backed up until it was against a wall, weak and tiring, their owner stood motionless upon some rickety steps waiting to draw his gun. Before he pulled his gun and the coyotes rushed, the bulldog broke his chain and the spine of the first coyote. He went for another, and seized its head in its jaws and clamped down, its teeth cracking through bone and brain and pelt and eyeballs and teeth, the blood striped the snow and we all howled and bayed, my dad, the owner, the dog, the little bulldog and myself like a pack of the very deceased. The owner pulled his gun and executed the last coyote, and then the bulldog. He said that once it had the taste he could never keep it. The little dog followed him inside. You can't believe it's real. You can't believe the directors and the writers and the musicians got it so right. In diners you really do nod along to Tom Waits or listen to 50's rock 'n' roll. You sit at the bar with men who have scarred hands, big boots and full beards who 'don't give a fuck about where you're from' but who just want to drink glasses of spirits. One, two, three, four – that's how he measures the drinks and the stoolies love him. The old songs are kept alive by places like these, as are old friendships and old flames. Men eating breakfast eat the same everywhere, with their backs hunched and one hand scooping – the other covering the plate like they're still in school cafeterias. Please make sure you lock the doors and windows. The weather is changing. There's an Indian kid with one eye who salts the car park. We say, they give you all the good jobs don't they, and he says, they sure do. He removes his scarf and he tells us that humans are killing mother earth and he says, this ain't cold, he says that he likes the cold, when he was young he used to swim under the ice. My dad says that every day you're vertical is a good day, he nods his head and carries on salting, whistling. At the town of Ulysses, my old man turns to me and says, imagine if we came out here a hundred years ago, the things we could do. We sit in a rare silence and stare at the snow on stone beaches and the vast continuum of fresh water, Finger Lakes, the little tributaries from the mountain bubble and trickle, muffled by the ice and moving as if every inch is a frontier to be conquered. The people that live here aren't like what you think, they love the land and care for it. The trees have been permanently affected by the wind, crooked spines and twisted manes of branches, they stand alone against the sweeping barrage. We leave the trees and enter prairies where the snow is dusted on the fields like flour on fresh bread. Geneva has old hotels and no visitors, huge murmurations of birds follow our truck, breaking in waves and moving with the free coordination of chainmail. Are you too heavy? There's no need to be ashamed of your weight. I used to do marathons but then I got an office job. Miles and miles pass, and then there is a barn with its middle boughs so sagged it reaches to the ground and we can't understand why it hasn't fallen in on itself. There is no split in the wood, it's just bent, as if God himself brought down his hand upon its back and

FOR STEVE

warped it in some terrifying show of power. We leave Lima and go to Leicester, Seneca Falls, and Lutterworth. This new road gives you the infinity view, straight as an arrow but undulated like some Dali picture, our heads are swivel mounted and we list everything we see. We say it out loud to offer it some permanence, so it doesn't remain some fleeting thought or point of interest, but something that is saturated in meaning and important. We move through Buffalo ghettos and there's not much to tell as it is exactly what you would expect. We drop the truck off and get a cab. Mr Ahmad, our driver, takes us to his home, it has shutters on the windows, a swing chair, and a white picket fence. When we cross the border and leave we tell him to enjoy his beautiful home, he says God bless you, I will. Niagara Falls makes me think of my great-grandmother, fourteen years old and the companion to six siblings, sitting atop a chest brimming with all their worldly possessions on a liner. She told me of the immense swells and the crashing of white and blue foam churning itself up and how Houdini was jettisoned off its edge. We are unimpressed with Canada and don't know what to expect from Toronto until we see it across the lake in a shimmering mirage of glass. You drive for miles and see nothing but suburbs and the last traces of industry until Toronto rises out of the ground like I imagine Mecca would. The sun reflects off glass towers and slides down, blinding us with threads of light, a monorail passes overhead in a warble and we weave between cars and wonder if Stan Lee has been here. Because if he hasn't, he should. We eat steak and drink a lot and I do little talking. Dad's talking, telling me that his theory of God is that people once worshipped dogs and we got the letters mixed round. He tells me about his inner chimp, saying that sometimes it's the right time to throw shit and sometimes you need to climb branches. We try and find dope but the shop is closed and instead there is a black girl with no front teeth who screams and begs me to go away and then we have a shouting match with a man whose chimp is visible. We pass out and leave the curtains open and so an orange light hums our eyes open, we eat fruit and the world is right, we drive to Nappanee to see my uncle. The house opposite my uncle's is full of drug addicts in various states of rehab. The girls could be so beautiful and the boys could be so strong but no one ever gave them the chance. It was minus nine last night and a girl lurched from the alley wearing nothing but a tee and dirty pants. Her legs were so thin that her feet pointed in and her knees stuck out. She was rattling from the gear and not the cold and I stood on the porch smoking and wanting to bring her into my chest and keep her in there until she's well. I'd do that, keep her in there, as many of them as possible – a menagerie of crackheads – until I couldn't keep them anymore. A Trojan horse of anguish and abuse, I'd lumber to the Nappanee court house steps and let it erupt from me like a fountain. It would sound like a bark and look like darkness and stop everything. It would be getting one back. My uncle has always sat in silence, a man of few words, but when everyone has gone to bed and the house creaks I hear him talking and talking and talking to his new wife. For us, he is somewhere beyond silence, absence. Propped up in bed he sits and reads, sighing – listening to us work on his house with saws and chisels. He will lay the book down across his legs and notice a train sounding three times as it approaches the town. He wears an ill-fitting yellow mask with a baldhead, my uncle, we all know he's under there somewhere and he hopes so too. Beneath the frustration at perpetual tiredness and anger at the injustice, which would see him sixty, and in love for the first time, with a new house and wife but with cancer invading every organ and an insurance company hungry at his heels. Stephen Knight is dying, after, there will be only two of us left.

    They have a very slight sense of humor, the Indians, he says. We went to the reservation earlier and bought hundreds of cigarettes for his wife, Dominique, who lights the next one without stubbing the other out. We made a deal with a wiry Indian youth for an e-cigarette loaded with dope. My dad talked at him until he was convinced that we weren't cops and we were just nuts. We liked each other, we talked over the bongs and suppositories. I asked him about the ginseng and he liked this – telling me that it was a myth that it all came from China and not the reservations, just cos it sounds funny, he says. I asked him about a jar with cash in, and a picture of two girls. Bone cancer, he said and so I put a five in. He nodded and turned, pulled out and showed us soft

FOR STEVE

resin that looked like pure tar, black lava, it wiggled from its tube as if with its own mind. We all stood in silence, my aunties, my dad, my cousin and I, watching it wiggle. Feral dogs roam the roads despite this reservation not being that poor. It's still poor enough for the young men to run drugs off the islands. Gangs of them drunk, reel in the snow and on the ice outside of bars looking for whites to fight, I don't blame them and I wish I could oblige them. Their house is not finished and is filled with yellowed worn furniture, brass handled and cut like shells. Dominique's grandmother bought it all in the 30's, in a market in Paris and you can smell it on it, and see how it was piled and bartered over. We have a barbeque in the snow, the house is ablaze with light and it stands out from the rest of the vacant row. A chrysalis of heat and light in pure white. My cousin Ethan is half Indian and overweight, he gets bullied by the refugees at his school and he's a good kid. His mother openly flirts with me, I'm quietly told that's just her way. We guzzle beer and wine and talk about what we can and finally we let my dad talk for us. I used to worry that we were all mad and now I'm happy for it. I sleep on the floor with my coat under my head and my boots on. The next morning Ethan tells me he doesn't know his dad and doesn't want to, I tell him that I have felt like that once. He says he's never had curry and he can't remember England. I tell him that he should come soon and he sits apart from us thinking. Dominique says my dad's not right, and I say who is, she recognizes it's not done him any harm apart from the swollen brain and the skin grafts and the broken noses. When we say goodbye to Steve we exchange the strongest of handshakes and the limpest of hugs. He stands on the porch in slacks and braces, his hands in his pockets and his eyes to a sky which is clear and with a sun that gets so hot that we can feel it on our faces and the boys fishing on the ice have to come in. We stop at a diner on the way back through the res and I think of all the things I should do. After coffee we stand outside and don't say much by way of goodbyes. Steve dies sometime later and we don't see where his ashes go. We know it was off a rock on an island, channelled down lanes over crisp water where salmon leap and big pines bud up. I imagine chanting, I imagine all the things that he was and wore. A beard and wool jumper, a pipe for many years and then cigars. Gliding down remote waterways and down inlets; lighting fires and sitting around them. Doing crosswords and reading. *Walking Death Valley* and finding South African separatists in Namibia. I think of chanting, I think of a train pipping three times and a dog's growl. But I don't think of this then, only where we have to go. Ethan takes me to one side and asks me if he can change his last name to Knight, I say that would be fine.

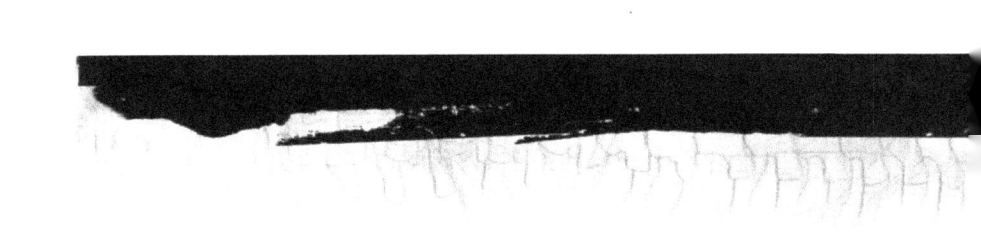

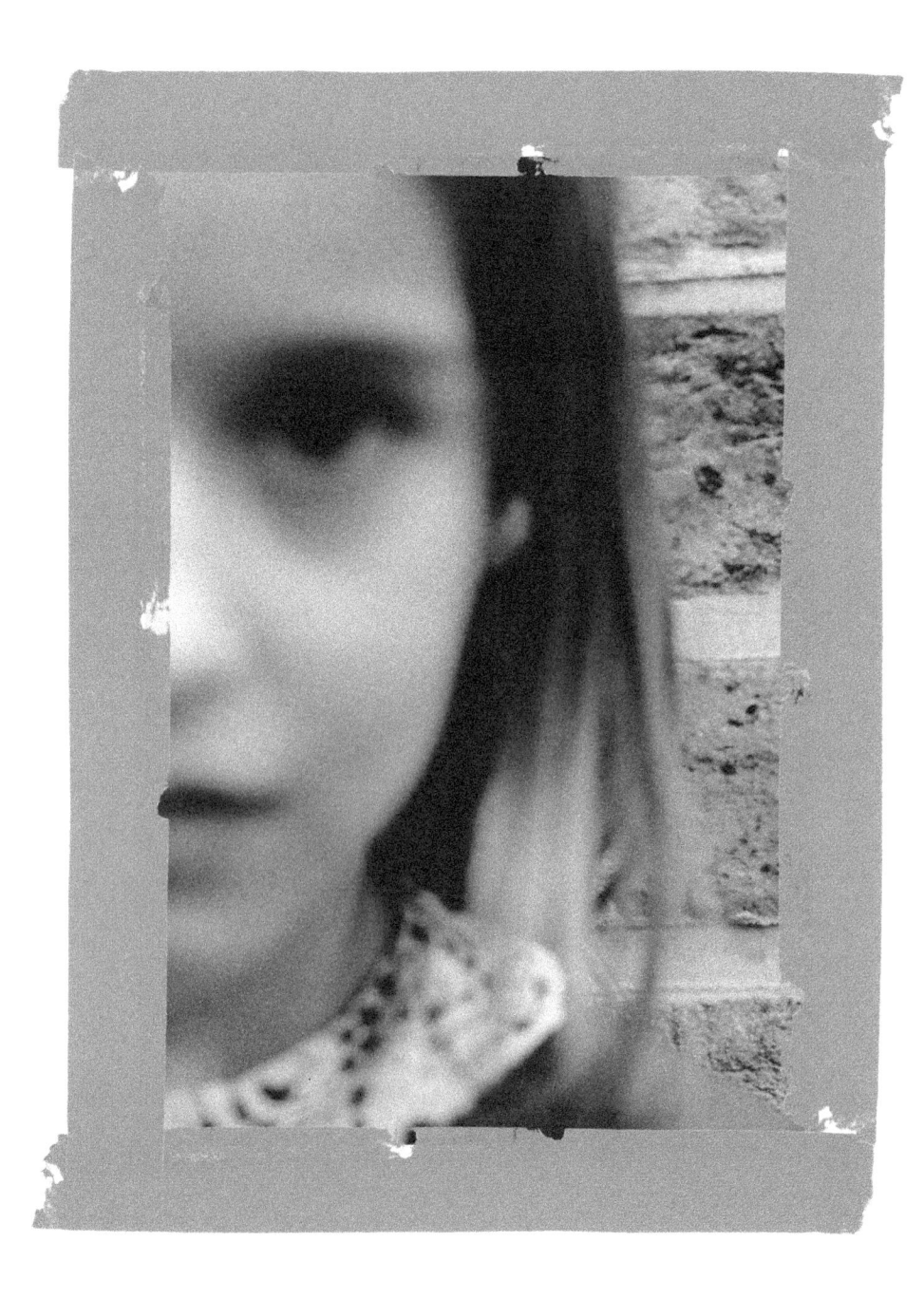

HILARY'S FEAST

by Sarah Longthorne

Erin didn't remember much afterwards. All she knew was that she'd woken in the ambulance, and the woman who called herself 'new mummy' – who Erin thought of as 'Laura' – had shaken her head as she spoke to the paramedic. 'Told me some "stranger" did it,' Laura said. 'But all I heard was a clattering across the kitchen floor. See, I'd only just got comfortable. The dishwasher at Smilie's broke today, and the baby was kicking, and on top of that I thought, "She's broken something." I was ready to lay the law, you know? Then I went in and found her with her arm dripping blood over my sink, and... I lost it. Not my fault, mind. Girl's been odd from the get-go.'

Erin had strained to see her arm. It was all in bandages, and on the cloth above her wrist was a blossoming red rose. The stranger had smiled at her from the foot of the trolley.

***

Erin awoke again in the hospital, and she was alone. She sipped some juice left by the bed and waited. Eventually, a nurse came by and told her she could soon go home, so long as she answered some questions first. The nurse asked about her past, and Erin said that she didn't remember much, except that one month ago a man had pushed her mother down the stairs. He was in all the photos, she said; perhaps that's how she recognised him. The nurse said nothing about Erin's scars.

There was silence on the drive home. Erin went to bed without dinner that night and Laura got drunk in the living room.

At fourteen, the stranger's visits became commonplace. She would come by early in the morning, and at awkward times when Erin was seeing friends or playing with Jamie, Laura's son, who'd been born with defects. Often, the stranger sang him to sleep.

'You can't come round when other people are here,' Erin said one night, sitting the stranger down on her bed. 'You always get me into trouble.'

'Other people like me,' the stranger replied. Her face curled into a smirk. 'Like me better than you.'

It was true; Erin's friends always had more fun when the stranger came by, and when she left, Erin could tell they missed her. So Erin nodded then – nodded down at her feet – and they never spoke of it again.

***

When Great-Aunt Hilary was dying, the stranger decided she would accompany Erin and Laura to the bedside. 'Been ages since I saw a dead person,' she said, gazing at the ceiling as Erin arranged her hair. 'Think she'll be all stiff and white?' The stranger wiped her expression, fell on her back, and performed her best impression of a corpse, which quickly cracked with laughter.

'She's not dead yet,' said Erin, ignoring her. 'She'll probably look very peaceful, though – when she goes, I mean. Least, I hope so. Not nice to talk about people like that.'

But Great-Aunt Hilary did not look peaceful. Wide, unfocussed eyes searched wildly in the ceiling. Her claw-like fists – sealed shut with arthritis – twitched against the duvet, remembering that once they could open. She tried to speak, but all that came from her mouth were parched 'muh' sounds.

As Laura and the girls stared down at the old woman, Erin imagined Great-Aunt Hilary as a bone table: an ornate, spindly frame draped with tissue for a tablecloth that sank into the hollows of her eyes and cheekbones.

The stranger folded her arms and grimaced. 'Dried up hag. Could take a feather duster between those legs.' Erin did not reply. The woman had supposedly taken ill when she was young and cut herself off from the family, claiming that she and all her blood were a tainted sort, possessed and cursed, and it was wickedness to allow it to continue. The only person she'd opened herself up to was Erin. Now time had worried away at her, and she was alone.

Erin looked closer at Great-Aunt Hilary, and this time she imagined that the woman on the bed was a feast that had never been eaten. The soup had gone cold, the bread was now stale, and the cheese was all green on the side. Erin pictured her own feast, untouched by all. She saw herself, an old spinster, holding out her pomegranate heart and breaking its skin with her nails to let the seeds tumble out like rubies.

As Erin stared, the old woman turned her head and smiled as if into a mirror. Her eyes drifted to the stranger and the expression faded. Her lashes glistened.

***

There was a great to-do about the inheritance when Great-Aunt Hilary passed. Erin was not of legal age, so anything owed her would go to Laura, who had set off early that morning to see the solicitor. A note on the fridge told Erin to walk little Jamie to school. The stranger walked beside them, trailing a stick across the railings like a xylophone.

'Old hag's death has got me wondering what sex feels like,' she mused, breaking the silence. Erin blushed. 'He's not deaf,' she hissed, covering the child's ears.

The stranger shrugged.

'He doesn't know what it means. If I said "fuck" he wouldn't know what it means. Doesn't know what anything means, the little frog.' The stranger rolled her eyes towards Erin. 'I bet it's amazing.'

'Laura says it hurts and you get diseases,' Erin looked around to check that nobody was listening.

'Even eating hurts if you do too much of it,' the stranger shot back. Erin choked back a laugh, then bit her lip and looked at her feet. When she raised her eyes, the stranger was glaring at her.

'Wanna end up like that shrivelled-up dead witch?'

'N-no,' said Erin.

'Then we gotta get moving,' said the stranger.

They arrived at Jamie's school. Erin bent down to muss his hair and kiss his face, but the boy stared blankly past her. She pinched his rosy cheeks and watched as he drifted into the building.

The stranger waited until they were walking again. 'Jake's sexy,' she said. 'Plus Rosie said he was really good and has a mouth that tastes like peppermint.'

'I don't like Jake,' Erin replied.

The stranger rolled her eyes. 'Tom? Still?' She paused, thinking. 'He's so quiet. It's like there's no one in.'

Erin shrugged. 'He's nice to me.'

'Fine, fine. Tom it is, as long as it's disgusting like a music video.' The stranger abandoned her stick and skipped ahead of Erin, touching every lamp post on her way.

When they got to class, the stranger wrote Tom a note and dropped it on his desk. His mouth dropped open, and his neck went redder than his pencil case. Erin put her head in her hands.

'It's embarrassing now, but at least you've done it,' said the stranger. 'Not gonna dry up like old Hilary.'

When all the students were packing up their belongings, Tom tapped Erin on the shoulder. She turned to look at him, and he, in turn, looked down at the desk. His face was like seeded bread behind his glasses. For a moment, neither of them spoke. With a glance at the gawking, departing students, he took her hand and led her around the side of the building.

Tom turned. 'Did you mean it?' he asked, grabbing her by the shoulders. 'This isn't a joke, right?' Without waiting for a response, he pushed his mouth into hers.

He was panting and wet-lipped by the time he let Erin go. 'I just didn't think you were like that,' he went on. 'Like, people say you go a bit hyper sometimes, and you can be a real fun time, but then you're always quiet, you know?'

He kissed her again, forcing her jaw open with his tongue. This time, Erin disentangled herself and stepped back. 'This is so hot!' Tom said, apparently to himself. He looked back at her. 'So, when? And where? Can we go to yours? My mum's super religious.'

Erin froze, pale and wide-eyed. The stranger stepped forwards and came between them. 'I know a place,' she said. Tom was grinning when he walked away.

Erin trailed the stranger to Great-Aunt Hilary's house: an expansive but empty almost-ruin on a weather-beaten hilltop just a half-mile out of town. 'Always thought he was so quiet,' she said. 'I didn't think he'd be like... like that.'

'I love it,' said the stranger. 'Don't you love it? How he wants you? How he'd do anything for you? You're like a goddess to him. He should worship you.'

They reached the front door, and Erin strained to see through the peephole. She tried the handle and pulled back. The stranger went around the side and tried a window. It opened, but her hand caught on the splintered wood. She laughed when she saw blood beading on her knuckles.

Tom arrived moments later wearing an ironed paisley shirt. He gawked. 'You broke in? Whose house is this?'

'It's just a house,' said the stranger. She took his clammy hand in hers, but he jumped away.

'You're bleeding!'

'Grow up,' she snapped. She grabbed Tom's hand and led him inside.

They stopped when they came to the first-floor bedroom, furnished with only a bare mattress. The room smelled of dust and stale perfume. There was no light other than the wan rods that speared through gaps in the boarded-up window, illuminating dust motes that span suspended in mid-air. Tom sneezed.

Erin positioned herself across the room from him and glanced up, her heart drumming dark blood to her forehead, neck, and ears. 'You've not done this before either, right? You're a... you're a virgin?'

He laughed, but his cheeks burned. 'Now you're all coy?'

Erin didn't respond. From the corner of the room, the stranger told Tom to strip.

He was a gangly boy, but he looked even skinnier without his clothes – like a disproportionate puppet on slack strings. They stood on either side of the bed, staring at each other. Tom shifted from one foot to the other. His hands twitched towards her like sunflower heads trailing the sun. 'Did you like it?' he murmured.

'Like what?'

'When... When I kissed you.' He blushed. 'Earlier.'

'Oh!' Erin blinked. She offered a smile. 'Oh. Yes. It was nice.'

A pause. 'Are you going to get naked then?' he asked.

Erin glanced down at her blouse. Her fingers trembled as she reached for the buttons. She looked up and caught the eye of a small painting of Great-Aunt Hilary atop the mantelpiece in front of a large, speckled mirror. Erin kept her eyes there as her clothes fell around her.

Tom licked his lips, which, Erin now saw, glistened beneath a fresh film of chapstick. His eyes were fixed on her breasts, and for the first time in her life, she considered that the body she'd thought of so functionally might not be appealing to other people. She crossed her arms over her tummy and fixed her gaze on the bed.

'What are all those pale marks?'

'I don't know,' said Erin. 'I don't... I don't remember.' She paused and looked towards the mantel. The portrait now seemed familiar in a secondary way, as if it held two faces instead of one. 'The man,' she said. 'The one in all the photos.'

There was a sigh. Across the room, the stranger got up and sauntered over to Tom. 'You're heartbreaking. Both of you,' she said, casting a smirk at Erin.

Tom's glasses skittered across the floorboards, and the mattress springs hiccupped under the weight of two bodies.

Erin watched. She stood there, holding herself, and looked on as the stranger took Tom's virginity. She saw the irregular, grunting awkwardness of it all. When she turned to the mantel, Great-Aunt Hilary and the man in all the photos stared back at her. The feast remained untouched.

The stranger left Tom sleeping when they finished. She smacked her lips against her forearm and dragged on her school trousers. 'You wouldn't have liked it,' she said. Then she left the room.

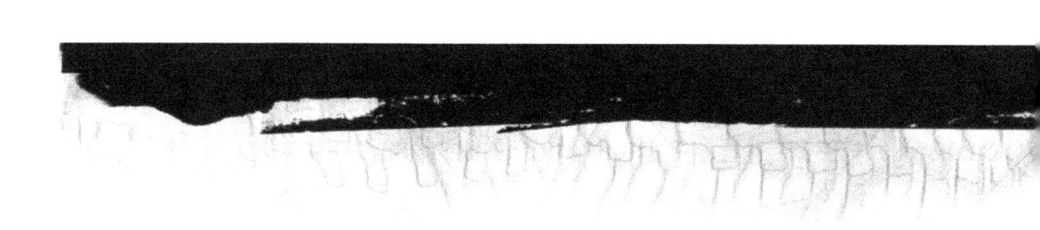

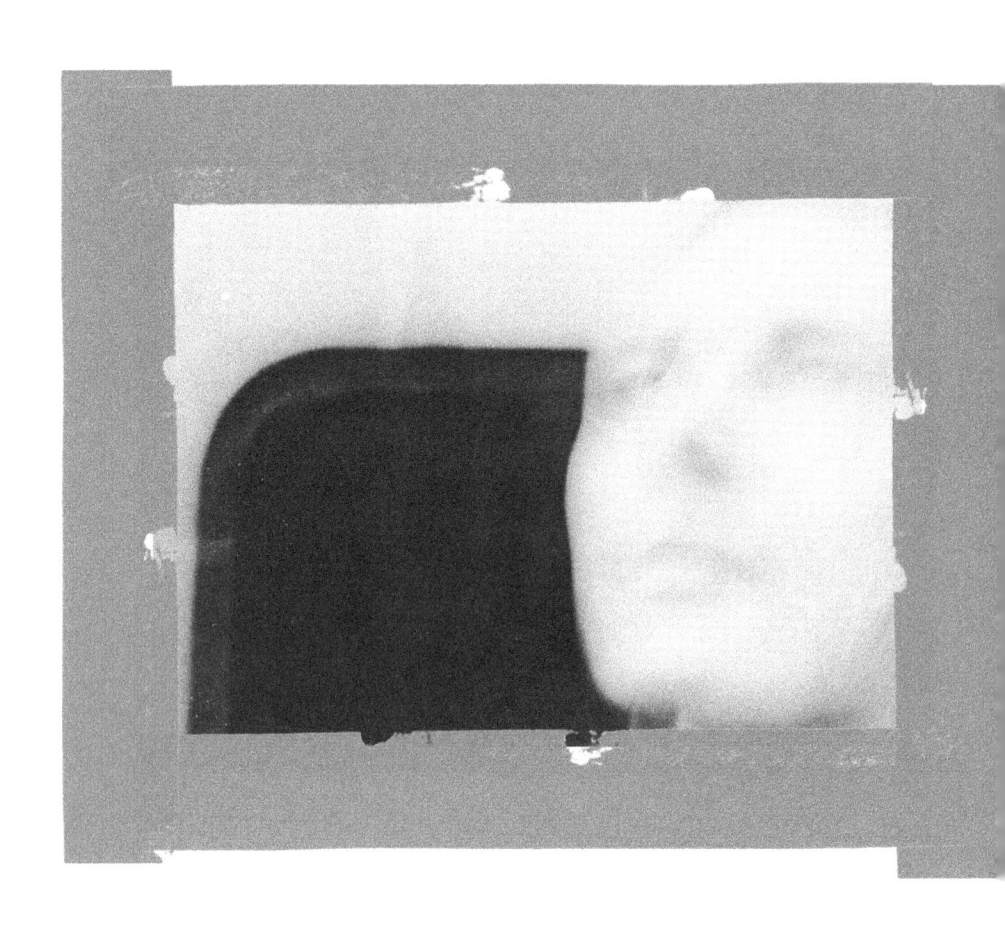

MY SPACESHIP

by Alison McCrossan

He hugs me so tight all I see are stars flickering in my eyes, and I get a whiff of pheromones that don't spark to mine. He's babbling as he breaks away, still holding me, and tilting back his head to look into my eyes. This is the direct opposite of a limp wet handshake, but has much the same repellent effect.

'Jesus loves you,' he says finally.

'No. The universe spits on me every day,' I say, wondering why I am entertaining a Bible pusher.

'I knew you were troubled the moment I set eyes on you.' He plonks down on his backside on the pavement and pats the space beside him, asks me my name. I sit. Why not? Nobody else in Cork will talk to me anymore. My deep-inside scars make me scowl. 'Jenny,' I say, the word funny on my tongue. I haven't said it in a while.

So, he touches my arm. 'It can't be that bad.'

So I tell him about my spaceship that I can't find.' '...and I've had to do the shittiest jobs on this world, Earth, just to survive... the worst?... A sex line operator. You have no idea how tedious people's fantasies are.'

He smiles kindly and rubs my shoulder. 'How about I help you find your spaceship?'

'Would you?' This is great, maybe Jesus is with this man and maybe he can talk to any Jesus-like being who lords it over my world. The name of my world I can't quite drag from my memory.

So we spend days searching for my spaceship.

'Why would you help me like this?' I say on the tenth day.

'I'm sick of my job.'

***

If he's sick of his job, he's sick of Jesus. I don't consider this a good omen. With every passing day and night spent in the woods my hope had grown that his Jesus would talk to my Jesus, a hope expanding like a new-born universe. Big Bang.

He's as lanky as a drainpipe that's come loose and is hanging from the wall, a little unhinged and a little lost. We're the same height – staggering for me at 6 ft 3. *Too tall for a girl. Too tall for a girl.* That's what the Earthlings say, but I never cared about that one – I mean how inane!

He's got big brown eyes with heavy lids and bags underneath. A symmetrical face though – humans like that, love that, it's the scientific marker of beauty. I have mapped his features diligently using an imaginary x-y axis and he'd be perfect to human eyes if he stood upright and used cream under his eyes – or slept until he felt refreshed; probably unable to sleep, like myself. He's starting to stink like me, a muskier male version of not washing. He looks less smooth now his white shirt is stained and creased, his smart black trousers need an iron, and his shoes for suits are in need of a polish. Bible pushers in this city tend to look the same, all good clean looks and dress. I like the dirt on him.

I hold his eyes now. 'Why are you sick of your job?' Not sure I want to hear; he's supposed to be helping me find my spaceship, not me helping him find himself.

He glances back at me with laden eyes.

So he says, 'It's a vocation, a calling, but–but–what can I compare my disappointment with it to, the loss of my desire to follow it? Losing a child – no, that would be presumptuous and I wouldn't know such a thing, and I don't think I'm that special. Okay, maybe I did once – once I believed I held a firm link to Jesus. That was egotistical maybe, deluded even. Faith is blind like having a child is blind; after all, for all the planning in the world and there's often not much planning involved, the child will turn out as the child will turn out.'

I nod, but I'm not entirely sure what he means other than he has lost faith; maybe that's enough. 'You need to restore your faith again,' I say. 'I need your Jesus to talk to my Jesus, or we might never find my spaceship.'

He smiles wearily and I notice flecks of blue in his irises. So I say, 'There's a bit of the sky in your eyes.'

He smiles bright now. 'What a lovely thing to say.' He looks up at the sky. 'Maybe that's where it's all at, the nature of things, the sea, the earth, the sky, and the universes extending beyond.'

'It is, it is, I agree, but we need your Jesus.'

He nods and smiles broadly. 'You want to hear the word. The problem is nobody else wanted to hear words about Jesus, and then the harder I tried to make people understand I just wanted the world to be a better place, the more they dismissed me, you see. What's wrong with wanting a better world?'

I want to cry for him. All the Earthlings I have met want a better world; they're just too consumed with survival and everyday concerns and a sense that it isn't within them or their place to ring in the change. The other Earthlings, the ones who don't want a better world, I have never met, though I have seen some on those broadcasts humans like to make about themselves and their concerns, starting wars and dishing out propaganda about money and deciding who should have it.

He looks like he's going to cry, head down, then he raises his face to look at me. 'So what's your world like?'

I shrug. 'Dunno. I can't find my spaceship so I can't get there.'

He opens his mouth to speak, gulps on air, and no words come forth.

I want to ask him why he never asked me this before, considering he thought I had clear memories of it, but I think I know why: he wanted to believe. Or did he? Nobody else ever believed me: the professionals (one or two) wanted to *help* me at first, feed me with drugs, lock me up in a unit until I became stable enough to make my way in the world, and go home here on Earth. *You're a nice lady, let us help you. You're intelligent, with so much potential.* Their idea of potential was very different to mine. I wanted real jobs, real relationships. I wonder, will his enthusiasm for travelling with me when we find my spaceship remain? Hopefully: he's an alright sort and good enough company, and we may be on a long journey through the universes.

***

On the twelfth day outside the city, he says, 'We need a metal detector. These woods are vast enough, and it's just a hunch you have that your spaceship crashed here.'

'My foster mother loved these woods. I know, the way she talked about them, that this is where she found me. She would say I was conceived here and giggle, but I know she's not my biological mother.'

His brow furrows. 'Was she cruel?'

'Oh dear God, no. Don't get me wrong, she was my mother in every sense, but she was an Earthling through and through. I am clearly not.'

He nods. 'We can get a metal detector online, and get it delivered to my address, but I gave all my money to the church last week, apart from rent and some pocket money, and I will run out of that in a day or two as well.'

'There is a debit card back at the house with a little money from the sex-line work. I lost the keys, and haven't been back there in a while, but we'll find a way in.'

His eyes widen like the sky opening up after a storm, 'You have a home?'

I bite down on my lip. Said too much. He'll view me differently. Worse, could he be like so many others, some of those who would *help* me, and see an opportunity for gain in the home I was bound to inherit and my meagre savings? Did he target me from the outset? 'Yes.' I continue with a lie, 'But I'm in the process of handing it over to an animal shelter, along with the money. There's no going back on that now.' I haven't much thought about what I should do with it when it becomes mine;

my only concern has been finding my spaceship. 'Where did you think I lived?'

'The streets first, then later, these woods – that shelter we passed.'

'I sleep under the shelter sometimes. Why are you helping me, honestly?'

He lowers his eyes, contemplates the mulch of brown-black leaf litter on the ground. 'I went along with it, not sure why. Maybe because I'm hopeless.' He glances up at me. 'Maybe because I'm so lonely.'

I read honesty in his tone, his body language and the blue flecks in his eyes. I glance up through the canopy of trees; the autumn sun is low and makes the sky yellow through the gaps, blending in with the edges of leaves, lighting on any remaining green. There is beauty in this world – why do I always forget that these days?

We go to my mother's house at the edge of the woods. It looks like Atlantis rising from a sea of coral reef. Flowers for every season; my mother taught me how to garden. I let the wild in when she died ten years ago, the natives and the aliens get along just fine to my eye, a staggering growth of weed and tree and bloom, vibrant colours from another place making no mockery of the more sedate Irish hues – no less lovely the interlopers say.

I find the debit card and we trek to the city streets, where we meander through bodies, hustlers, preachers, political cause campaigners, until we find the internet cafe and purchase a metal detector.

***

We settle back into the woods for the night as we have done for the previous two weeks. The metal detector is due to arrive at the Bible pusher's flat in the morning. I call him by his birth name, Sean, now. He told me that when he joined the church first he took the name Paul and hasn't been called Sean in a long time.

Sean asks me about my mother. What should I tell him? I was a burden to my mother during her life. Considered unwell, unstable, labelled mad, dismissed by this society; I was good enough to exist here on Earth but not good enough to function. Put up with. She bore the brunt of this expectation placed on me, and that inevitably I took upon myself. I wanted to make a place for myself here on Earth, but it was too obvious that I didn't belong. Then she disappeared twelve years ago. Two years after that, I accepted she was dead, and I would never see her again. The Gardaí files on her case remain open. He may even have heard about her on the news, but there are so many missing people cases these days and other dismal, sad, outrageous news stories, will he remember? Would I remember the faces of all those missing people on the news if it hadn't happened to me? To my mother?

Did she walk away?
Was she taken away? Please don't let her have been taken away.
Please don't let her have walked away.

Eventually, I say, 'She was amazing. That sounds dull. How can I convey to you in mere words what she was like, her spirit, her essence, her presence?'

He smiles gently, 'You're doing a nice job so far.'

She wouldn't have walked away, not in her senses.

I shake my head. 'She was more than a mother; she was my best friend too. That's all I can say.'

He nods.

'What about you?' I say. 'You say you are lonely.'

'I have family; my parents are alive. They live in Dublin. My sister too. I never felt close to them, then when I joined the Church – well, they said it was a con job, the Church just wanted me to recruit and bring in more money for them.'

'Sounds like they may have been right; you say you gave all your money to the church.'

He places his head in his hands and mutters, 'I need to believe. I need to believe.' He looks back at me now, with fire in his eyes. He's curling his fingers into his palms tightly. He's raging. 'Don't say that.'

'What about...' I soften my tone and smile. 'What about friends, a woman? Or a man – a partner, I should say.'

'Separated after a year. She says I am cold. I'm not cold, I'm not. I just find it hard to express myself. My boy hardly knows me.'

My heart is beating hard. Am I in danger after all? A woman knows things in an intimate relationship, such as if their partner is a cold fish.

He's red in the face, scratching at the skin on his cheek. He stops abruptly. 'I'm scaring you. Don't be scared of me. Don't be fucking scared of me.'

He's making my heart beat faster. I'm planning my escape: pretty much to run as fast as I can through the woods. He's a man but he's not as fit as me and isn't used to finding places to hide in these woods.

He lies down abruptly and within seemingly impossible minutes he is snoring.

I need help to find my spaceship.

***

I sleep with a rock in my hand and when I wake he is cooking sausages and eggs over the fire. I taught him how to set a fire and he whooped like a child the first time he succeeded in lighting it.

I keep the chatter light; he hardly talks at all but smiles as he hands me breakfast. I'm struck once more by those blue flecks in his eyes; the fire seems to spark them in the early half-light, like stars, hot as hell, but with a cool aspect set by sheer distance.

Thinking about my world now, I eat in silence. Why are my memories of it so dim yet so concrete? It feels like a past life; I sometimes wonder if it is and if I was born into this life and this world after all. But somehow I know my spaceship crashed and dumped me here; my dreams about that machine and my brief existence before the crash are too vivid to be anything other than certain. Nobody understands or believes, but that's okay. I'm not even sure Sean believes. I know, as sure as I bleed and on this planet the colour is red, as sure as this planet has one sun that rises every morning and sinks every evening, as sure as the moon pulls on this planet, influential and magnificent, sound and stable.

'I'm sorry,' he's saying. 'I know I scared you. Please don't be scared of me.' His eyes are earnest; his smile is kind. I'm not exactly the queen of expression myself these days.

***

So we collect the metal detector and begin to scan the earth in the woods.

'How long have you been searching for your spaceship?' he says.

I think about this; I'm not sure. My memory is a strange beast, always letting me down, confusing me with half-images, smells, sounds that promise much revelation but never deliver. 'I feel like I have been in these woods forever.'

'But you lived in the house once?' he says.

The metal detector bleeps and he sweeps it across a wide area. Bleep bleep bleep. 'Were you happy in the house?' He's talking but examining the earth.

I think and I think.

He lets me think, turning off the metal detector.

'I was, yes. Until my mother disappeared.'

He looks at me now eagerly. 'Disappeared? What do you mean? Do you think she went off in a spaceship?'

'No. Of course not. She's a missing person. Nobody knows what happened to her, but she wouldn't leave. She was taken.'

'By your – people?'

'No – I mean – I never thought of that. I always presumed a monster, I mean a human monster. You know what I mean.'

He nods.

I want to scurry away and hide. How many times have I heard footsteps in these woods, a branch snapping, or the rustling of leaves, and run for cover from the monster?

He scratches at the dirt with his foot. 'Do you think this might be your spaceship, buried here?'

'What are the chances?'

He's looking forlorn. 'We'll never get it to lift-off out of here, even if we figure out the controls.'

'No,' I say.

I must have always known about my spaceship, but I would never have taken off in it while my mother was here.

MY SPACESHIP

'No,' he says.

So, he puts his arms around me and holds me tight, stars sparking in my eyes. His Jesus has spoken to mine.

'I may never find her,' I say lowly. *Not in this life.*

His eyes are filled with sadness, tinged with regret, and the blue specks seem to have faded out.

'But your wife and your child and even your biological family can still be found,' I say.

Blue flecks simmer in his eyes once more.

So, I scratch the words *'goodbye for now, Mum'* into a spiralling horse-chestnut tree shadowing the site of the spaceship.

But, Mum, please come home. Please.

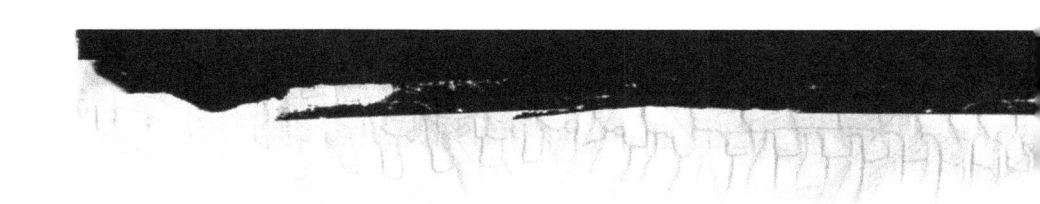

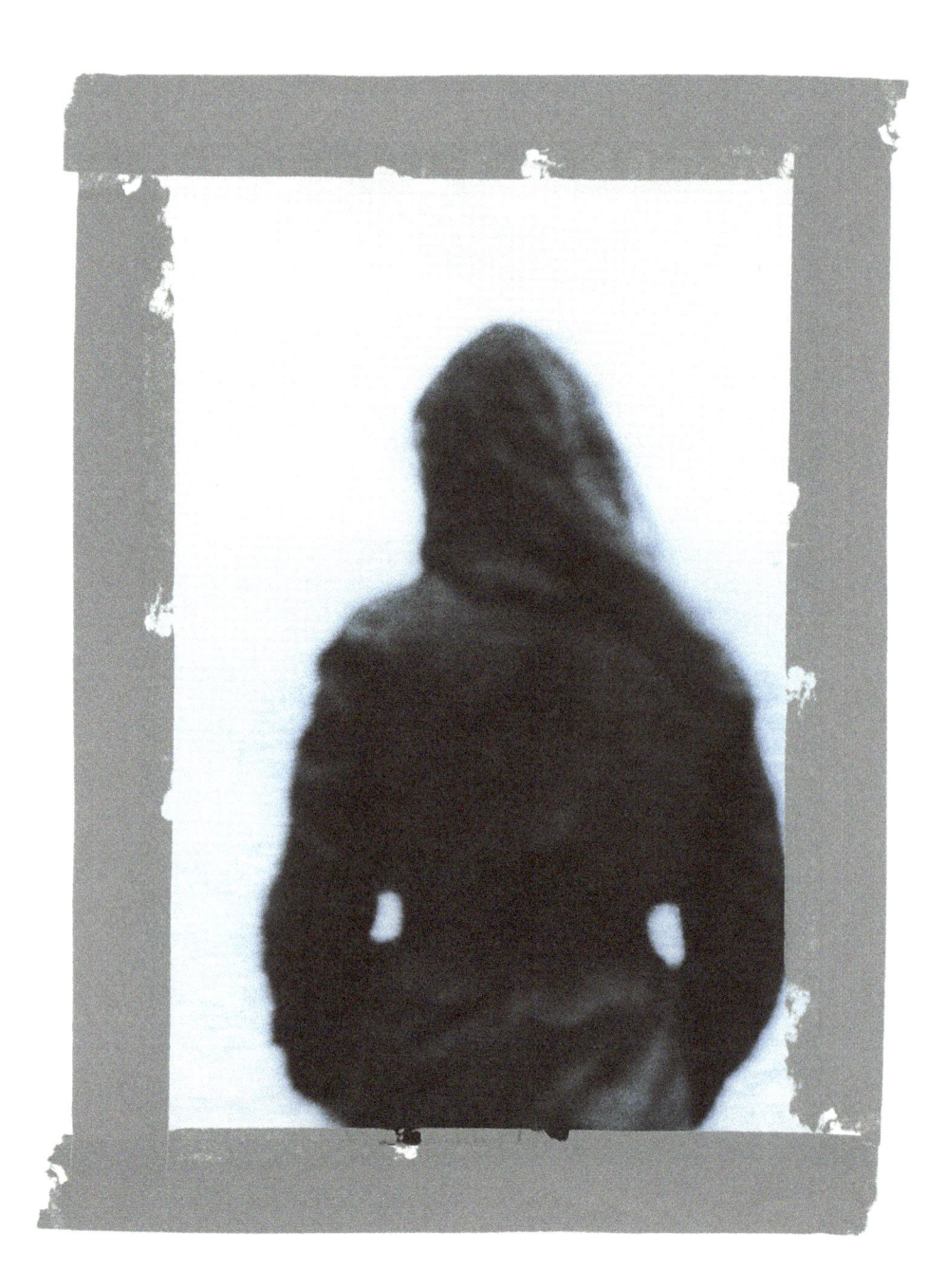

FLIGHT

by Roland Miles

I am strapped into the rear of the car, my little brother in the adjoining seat. We are stationary, facing downwards on the incline of the drive, looking out on to the field in front of the house. Below that is the aerodrome. The field is called the Denshawe – field of the Danes. I look at the back of my father's head as he starts the car. My mother reaches back and pats my arm. There is a moment of confusion when I am told that we are going to the airport. We watch through the wall-high window as my mother's plane takes off. My father is left behind. I am left behind. My brother is returned to us a year later. My mother who is not a mother now lives in America, and sends gifts which arrive late. I have not seen her for 1431 days.

Ours is a silent house. Our neighbour looks in each day. She stays until my father's return from work. I sit in the garden, looking down the hill, watching the planes. She comes out and sits alongside me. She wears a necklace, beads in several shades and sizes, mismatched, strung together. 'I found them one by one,' she says. 'They were dropped on the road, just down there,' she says, pointing.

'Are they Viking?' I ask, thinking of the Denshawe.

'Saxon,' she says. 'People have walked this path for thousands of years. Just like the litter down by the side of the road, so their debris was dropped as they went by. Small clues that they were here once. The stories they could tell...'

'Are they valuable?' I ask.

'I offered them to the museum but they have hundreds so I had them made up like this. My little connection with the past.'

My brother sits upstairs by his window, head down at his computer. He has the best room in the house. 'For his telescope, he needs a clear view,' my father said. From there he can see down the hill, over the airfield and out across the sea. At night, you can see the car lights shimmering past, and the winking of the beacons both on the airfield and at the port.

When my father comes home, I go upstairs. I knock at my brother's door but there is no answer. I go in. He is absorbed, putting the telescope up very carefully, laying the lens on to the bracket, securing it precisely and adjusting the various dials until he is completely satisfied. He likes to clean it. Each week, he dismantles the whole mechanism, polishing the lens and mirror, dusting the tube and buffing the white enamel on the outside. He will not allow anyone to help him. He knows what he is doing. 'Good night,' I say.

The air show draws large crowds in the summer. We can watch from the house, high above. 'Let me see,' I say to my brother. He steps reluctantly aside. 'It is a Sopwith,' I say. I recognise it from the guide he has on his desktop. I can see the roundel on the wing, and move the telescope very gently to the right. I can see the pilot's head, the leather straps and buckles on his leather helmet, his large nose. I am over a mile away and I can see all this detail. 'Look,' I say. 'You can even see the colour of his eyes.' He does not respond, pushes me aside and takes up his position again behind the lens. I do not try to look again. It is his telescope.

I stand in the garden. It is quiet once again at the airfield. I stare down across the expanse of the Denshawe. The cars steal past, nose to nose. My brother will be looking up at the stars tonight. Our neighbour calls out. 'I am going now. Your father is in his study.'

They burn back the stubble. The ground blackens in an almost even line across the field. The sun sets lower in the sky.

FLIGHT

I look over my brother's shoulder. A film plays on his screen. A de Havilland flies across the airfield and the camera follows it in a jerky motion. The focus is pulled and the camera plays over the airshow crowd. I see their mouths moving, hands raised in applause, captured in time. The picture changes abruptly to the control tower and I see a face beneath a cap, a mouth behind a microphone. 'You rigged the telescope to the webcam,' I say. My brother lays a hand on my arm and motions me to move. He pushes a button. The film speeds up. He stops it when he is satisfied.

It is an ordinary car, a Ford, paint scratched on the driver's side, the one which faces the camera. I can even read the number plate. In the driver's seat is a man, or a boy. A girl, in a red coat, throws her suitcase into the back and climbs into the front seat. I know her face. Everyone knows her face. The boy puts his left arm across her shoulder and pulls her towards him. She allows herself to be drawn to him. They do not kiss, but press their foreheads together.

I hit the return button and watch it replay. She is smiling. It is almost a still frame but for a slight flicker. I am there with them in that moment. She moves her hand: 'Let's go'. He nods. I see the smile on his lips and in his eyes. They move off, joining the flow of traffic. The camera holds on the space where they have been. The screen goes to black.

'We should say something,' I say. My brother raises his finger to his lips. He selects the file and presses 'delete'. Beyond the window, the long lights of cars flicker over the ploughed ridges of the Denshawe as they disappear into the night.

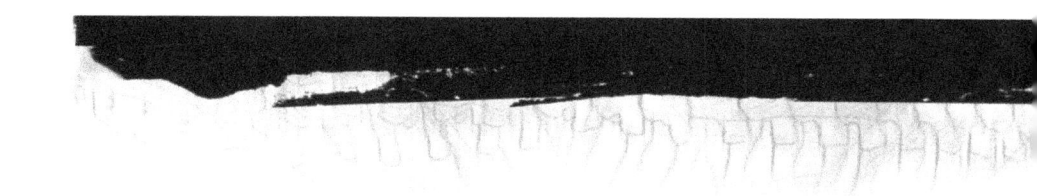

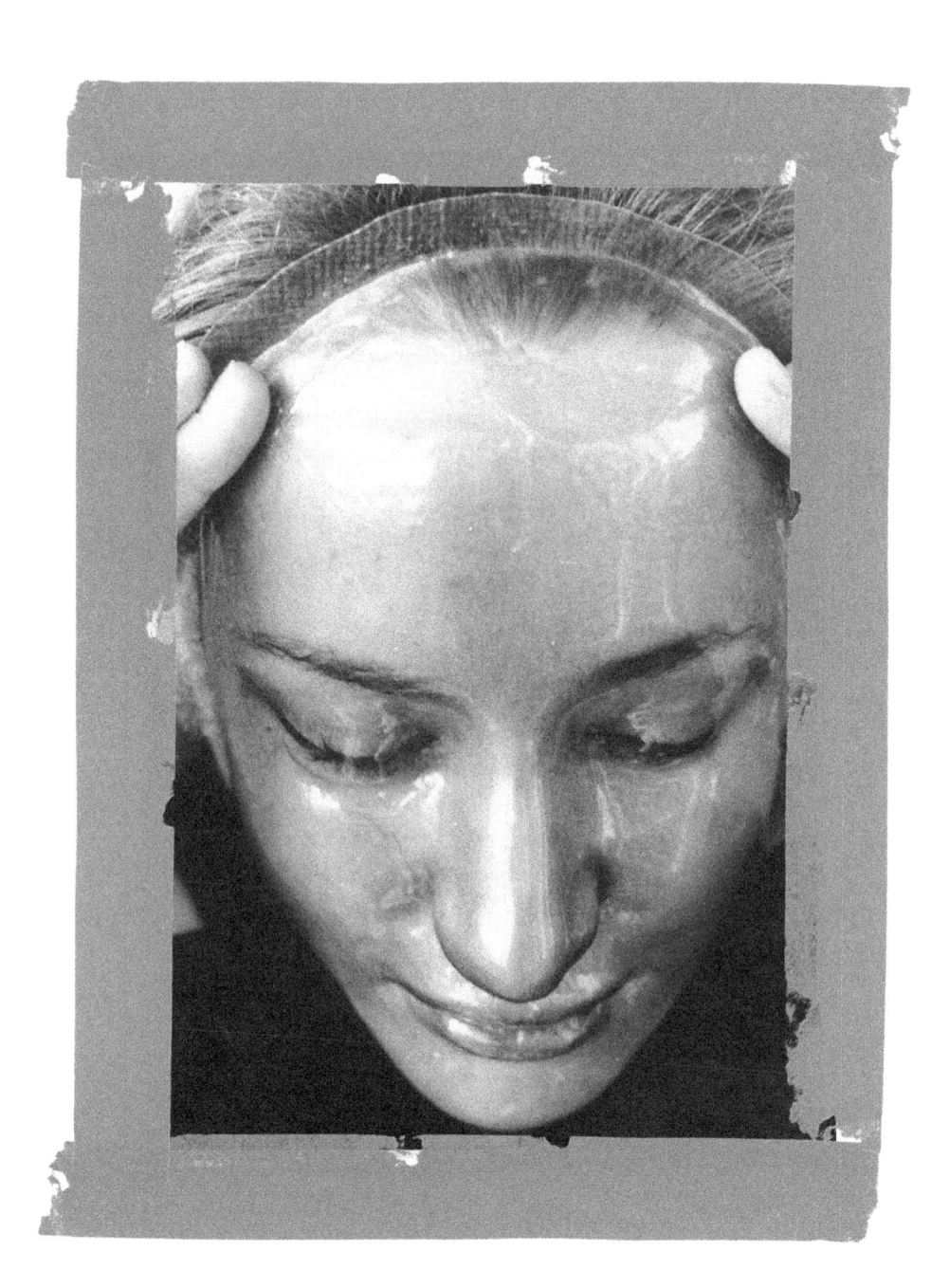

FINE NOW

by Diane L. Miller

Even before the puppy had been poisoned, Ellen knew it would be a nuisance. It had been one of those days when she contemplated sticking her hand in the office shredder to distract herself from the constant pain in her head, if only for a moment. She looked forward to lying down in a darkened room. A pet was the last thing she needed.

The children found the puppy dumped near the playground, and her husband, David, told them they could keep it.

Ellen had not had a chance to shut the door before the ambush started. At first, double vision from the migraine made Ellen see two mutts; one was bad enough. She told her pleading children that they would need to take it to the pound tomorrow. Chrissie and Tom promised they would do everything to take care of the puppy. Walk it, train it, wash it, clip its nails.

Chrissie wept and clung to the puppy even harder as it squirmed in her tight grip. Her tears were so lavish, they stained the collar on her polo neck shirt.

'I will take care of her! Honestly!' Chrissie cried in protest, rubbing her cheek against the puppy's head and kissing it. 'I will feed you good food, Sparky.' Chrissie scratched behind its black, floppy ears, which pricked up as if she had pressed a lever.

'Sparky's a stupid name,' Tom said.

'You can't name it because we're not keeping it,' Ellen said.

The children retreated to their rooms upstairs. From the kitchen, Ellen could hear Chrissie shout: 'I hate Mom. She's horrible!' When Chrissie slammed her door, the wall downstairs vibrated. Ellen sighed at the house's cheap new-build construction.

David, who had been in the home office, shuffled into the kitchen. He rubbed the wavy chestnut hair on the top of his head and glanced sheepishly at Ellen.

Ellen couldn't bear to look at him and turned away when she spoke. 'Can you get the kids dinner? I need to lie down,' she said.

As Ellen climbed the stairs to her bedroom, Chrissie's weeping and complaints grew louder. The dog yapped and whimpered in response.

After taking her migraine medication, Ellen showered and got into her pyjamas although it was not yet 8pm. The visual disturbances and pounding had dulled, leaving a constant hum of pain that clouded her thought. It felt as if her brain had swollen too big for her skull, like an overcooked boiled egg.

Ellen had lived with celiac disease all her life, as far back as she could remember. Since her diagnosis – finally – two years ago, she had been extremely careful. She and David used to eat out weekly, just the two of them; now, they rarely did. When she started bringing her lunch to work, it was clear: the cross-contamination had to be from home. Initially, David promised to keep the house gluten-free, but it gradually crept back in.

The bedroom door creaked open and David tiptoed in to get changed for the gym.

'What were you thinking?' Ellen's muffled voice strained under the covers.

'They're so excited. It's a cute puppy.' David switched on his bedside lamp.

Through squinted eyes, Ellen watched David pull sweatpants over his scrawny legs. 'There's no way we're keeping it,' she said.

'Let the kids have a little fun. Why do you have to be such a sourpuss about these kinds of things?'

Fun. Ellen wasn't sure what this was. David talked about fun like it was a destination, a cruise that some people took through life.

He didn't wait for her to reply before adding, 'It's a classic part of childhood, roaming around with your dog.'

'They don't roam far from TVs or video games,' Ellen said. 'I guarantee in a month they'll claim they're coming down with polio just to avoid walking the dog around the block.'

'This will get them running around more,' David said. 'Tom certainly needs to.'

'I can't manage taking care of a dog on top of everything else. It goes to the pound tomorrow.'

Over the following days, the children and David wore Ellen down. Chrissie and Tom bathed the puppy, walked it, fed it, trimmed its nails, gave it chew toys and treats, brushed it, and even cleaned up after its accidents. David bought it expensive gluten-free dog food because it claimed to be better for its health.

After a month, Ellen was surprised that the children's interest hadn't waned. She lounged in a deckchair, watching the puppy romp in the backyard with the kids. With the dog yapping and Chrissie's incessant chatter, Ellen found it hard to relax. She closed her eyes, trying to focus on the echoing drill of a woodpecker nearby.

Tom laughed and said, 'Aren't you cute, Sparky!' Ellen opened her eyes, astonished that her teenage son was calling something cute.

There was nothing cute about the dog. It was smelly, noisy and not much use. When she worked from home, Ellen fed the dog and let it out in their fenced backyard until its barking threatened to annoy the neighbors. Mostly it just chewed garden toys and the hose. Otherwise, it would sit in the kitchen slobbering over a toy or staring dumbly at Ellen while she typed at the table.

Chrissie clapped her hands as the puppy sprayed Ellen's snowdrop anemones and said, 'Good Sparky.' Chrissie rubbed the dog's ears and gave it a biscuit.

'Make sure it doesn't pee on the flowers again,' Ellen said. 'Or dig them up. I spend a lot of time trying to make everything look nice.'

Chrissie rolled her eyes. Her maturing face had grown awkward and angular, like a baby bird's. 'Sparky's not doing anything,' Chrissie said.

'There's already a dead patch in the corner.' Ellen stood up and walked back into the house. She had exhumed herself from bed early to clean, and already the kitchen was a mess. The children and David had not cleared up after breakfast. It looked as though the Pillsbury Doughboy exploded a suicide vest in the kitchen. Last week, she even found a breadcrumb in the coffee maker's water.

***

It wasn't until they were on the low road parallel to the lake that Ellen realized she had forgotten to make herself a sandwich. David had been busy getting the new buoys for the sailboat ready, Tom was preparing the fishing tackle and Chrissie needed to organize the dog's provisions. Ellen had barely finished making their sandwiches, using catering gloves, when David started beeping the horn in the driveway, eager to get out on the lake while the sun was still shining. It was too late to go back home now, and she was unlikely to find anything to eat at nearby convenience stores.

Once they unpacked and David tied up the buoys, Chrissie deposited the dog on deck. It stumbled drunkenly and whimpered, nails clacking against the boards. The lake was calm but the others clambering in rocked the boat. Chrissie picked up the dog and cuddled it. 'Poor baby,' she laughed. Chrissie sat with the puppy upright, facing out like an infant in a sling and exposing its white furry belly crested with limp curls. The dog's alert head darted around, then it gnawed at Chrissie's leather friendship bracelets.

Over the past week, the puppy had chewed Ellen's new loafers, rendering them unsightly and unwearable, the corner of a sofa cushion, David's sneakers and Tom's baseball glove. It disembowelled several of Chrissie's stuffed animals including her favorite, Ugly Monkey. Despite being nearly eleven, Chrissie was inconsolable about the mauling until Ellen restuffed it. Ugly Monkey now had a dark brown felt patch like a burn scar amid its matted fur.

Last night, the puppy howled at 3am for about twenty minutes. Ellen worried about the neighbors but was too tired to get out of bed. David slept through it, as he had when their babies woke up for feeds. It was like having a malevolent child in the house.

'Since there's not a lot of wind, can we just use the engine?' Ellen asked. 'We'll get there twice as fast.'

'But it will be half the fun,' David said. He kept the sails up, drifting more than sailing toward Apple Island. Ellen reflected that they could have swum faster to the fishing spot.

When David proposed buying a second-hand sailboat, Ellen didn't object. It would be a good way to spend family time and the kids could learn to sail like David had growing up. In reality, she resented having to jibe and tack. Leisure was not supposed to involve work. Cold winds made her bones ache even more than they already did. Instead of enjoying the serenity of being out on the water, Ellen spent the time thinking of all the things she should be doing but never had time for because she was constantly sick and exhausted. These tasks taunted her – a physical manifestation of her illness. The list was long and, she had to admit, she seemed to be the only one who cared.

Tom dropped a fishing line in the water as they sailed, a trickle of sweat running down his neck. The sun was out, and the lack of breeze made it feel hotter.

Nesting in a bed of old towels that they used to dry their seats, Sparky dozed, lulled by the gentle movements of the boat. The children ate their sandwiches. Ellen had a few handfuls of potato chips then set the bag down on the seat while she ate a banana. Tom stuck his hand in the bag and shoved some chips in his mouth.

'Did you at least dust the breadcrumbs off your hands?' Ellen asked. Tom shook his head, his mouth still full. He leaned over the side of the boat and dipped his hands in the water before drying them on his shirt, then grabbed some more chips.

Hunger crept over Ellen. Although she knew she should not risk eating more chips, she couldn't resist.

The wind picked up, blowing the boat, at long last, toward the banks of the island. Greasy-looking clouds now obscured the sun.

Having left her sweatshirt in the car, Chrissie started complaining about the cold. She was a marathon champion of whiners, and Ellen could not bear a display now. If Ellen had whined like Chrissie, even though in retrospect her illness had given her good reason to, her mother would have slapped her.

Ellen rubbed her temples, trying to suppress the violent pain taking hold. The cool wind and rocking boat only added to Ellen's misery and regret at her lack of self-control.

As the boat picked up, the dog woke and bolted from one end of the deck to the other, barking excitedly. A jaunty navy handkerchief with white anchors flapped around its neck as it ran. Ellen shut the door to the below deck to shorten its track. The children laughed at the dog's command of the ship. 'Sparky's a natural sailor,' Chrissie said. 'She loves the boat.'

Chrissie poured bottled water into a small bowl for the dog then handfed it gluten-free kibble. 'I can make Sparky sit. Sit, Sparky.' Chrissie pushed the dog's backside down. The puppy continued to sit in expectation of a treat. Its tail thumped the deck like a metronome. 'Did you see that, Mom?'

Ellen nodded mutely though she had her eyes closed.

As they approached Apple Island, the dog scrambled up to the bow of the boat, watching the ducks and geese migrating north in formations. The birds taunted the dog with their flight, remaining forever out of grasp. The children laughed at the puppy's ferocious barking, as though it were a toddler threatening destruction.

When they anchored, and David and Tom got out their fishing reels, the dog would not stay quiet. A heron sat atop a buoy, and in the island's maple and ash forest beyond, chicks perched provocatively in a rookery. David and Tom implored Sparky to stop. 'Maybe we should move away from the birds,' Chrissie said.

'Ellen and Chrissie, why don't you make yourselves useful and pull up the anchor?' David asked.

'Can we just go back?' Ellen said. 'I know it's a pain, but I'm really not feeling well.'

David looked at her like she had spoiled the trip. 'Again? I thought the doctor said you're fine now.'

'He said I should be fine if I can avoid cross-contact.' Ellen paused as she did not want to make Tom feel guilty but added, 'I think I may have been glutened from the chips.'

'Can't you just lie down below deck for a while?' David asked.

Ellen and Chrissie lifted anchor, and David sailed east before dropping it again. Ellen went below deck to curl in a fetal position on the small, cushion-covered berths. She would try to hold the shit in, not relishing the thought of sanitizing the slop bucket when they got home, among all the other things she needed to do.

Ellen closed her eyes; not long afterward, she heard a splash then a shriek from Chrissie. Thinking that Chrissie fell in, Ellen jumped up from the berth. But when above deck, she saw that Chrissie was leaning over the boat's edge yelling, 'There she is! She's going to drown!'

'She's doing the doggy paddle,' Tom said. 'Like dogs do. Hence the name.'

Sparky paddled closer to the boat. David leaned over and picked the puppy up by its kerchief. For a brief moment, Ellen thought: *Too bad it didn't go under.*

'Stupid dog.' David laughed and shook his head.

'What happened?' Ellen asked.

'She just jumped in like she wanted to swim,' Tom said. 'There's no reason to make such a big deal about it.' Tom shot a look at Chrissie.

Sparky shook the water off, flecking them in the face. Its curly black hair, still dripping and matted, looked like a bad home perm.

'We need to get Sparky a life jacket too,' Chrissie said.

David looked at his watch. 'Let's go back,' he said. 'It looks like we've had enough fun for today.'

***

Although they had been giving the dog plenty of water – food was a bad idea at this point – its head shrank into a dried-out apple, and its eyes sank into its skull. It had aged years in a matter of days.

When the vomiting and diarrhea first started, Ellen wanted to take it to the vet's immediately but capitulated to David's protests that everything would be fine in a day or two. Aside from her disgust, Ellen feared for her carpets. By the second day, when the dog's emissions came in constant waves, Ellen stuck it outside while she worked. It sprayed her flowers with vomit and shit, but Ellen no longer cared if it meant she didn't have to clean it up. She could just hose everything down. After a few hours, she found the listless dog lying on its side in the sun, shivering. The white patch on its belly had grown darker. She brought it food and water and moved it under a shady maple tree. A cardinal landed on a nearby branch, but the dog, dazed, didn't notice. When David and the children came home, they protested that Sparky had been outside all day.

'That's not very empathetic,' David said.

'I'm meant to be working from home, not nursing a sick dog,' Ellen said.

Once they brought the dog inside, the vomiting and diarrhea started anew. The children gagged and refused to clear it up. David made a great show of wiping the kitchen floor then mopping it with disinfectant.

On the third day, David helped Chrissie make a little bower from shrub cuttings under the maple tree, where they put several bowls of water and some kibble before they all left for work and school. When Ellen and the children returned home late in the afternoon, the dog hadn't moved, and diarrhea had pooled in the grass behind it. The dog lay on its side, its flank pulsing with rapid, shallow breaths.

Chrissie hosed the dog down and brought it into the kitchen, water dripping onto the floor tiles.

Ellen couldn't understand why, after several days, the dog seemed to be getting worse. She looked at it lying on a bed of old towels near the back door. The dog shivered uncontrollably and stared stupidly into space.

It was no state to be in, Ellen thought.

'Did it eat something it shouldn't have?' Ellen asked.

'She's always trying to eat things that people drop on the street, like pizza slices,' Tom said.

'Where have you ever seen pizza slices lying around?' Ellen asked.

'You'd be surprised. People leave all sorts of things in the park.

FINE NOW

Someone keeps leaving whole slices of bread.'

'That's probably meant to feed the ducks at the pond,' Ellen said.

Chrissie's face crumpled. 'I forgot. When I took her for a walk near the playground, I let her off the leash for a while. When I found her, she was eating some green bread.'

'You mean moldy bread,' Tom said.

'How much did it eat?' Ellen asked.

'I don't know,' Chrissie said. 'When I saw her, she was eating a slice, but it didn't look like she had that much.'

On hearing this, the dog appeared to try and represent itself, drawing up onto its knees. All of a sudden, it trembled and fell over on its side, making a dull thud against the floor. Its eyes were glazed and staring; its jaw champed and foamed at the corners; its legs paddled rigidly in slow motion, as if it were dreaming of drowning. A trickle of feces pooled on the kitchen tiles.

Ellen gently wrapped the disoriented dog in a towel and bundled it into the car. As they drove to the vet's, Chrissie wept in the backseat, clinging to the limp bundle of fur in her lap. 'Is she going to die?'

'I don't know,' Ellen said.

As she carried the dog from their distant parking spot down the town's main street, foot traffic steered clear, as though Ellen were an unwashed homeless person; the dog's stench preceded them. The vet was not optimistic; the bread mold had released poisonous mycotoxins in its gut. Its kidneys were starting to shut down.

Later that evening, the vet nurse called to tell them that Sparky was unlikely to last 24 hours. Neither of the children wanted to go to school the next day. Tom, she suspected, feared welling up and losing face among his friends. Ellen had to physically put Chrissie, guilt-stricken and heartsick, onto the bus.

Mid-morning, the vet rang Ellen to say that the dog seemed to be pulling through and would need to stay in a few nights to recover. The first thing Ellen thought was: *Too bad*. Then: *That's a grand gone*.

That evening, Ellen took Chrissie and Tom to the vet's for a visit. While the children consoled the dog, the vet informed Ellen that it had recovered only partial kidney function.

'Should we put it to sleep?' Ellen asked the vet.

'No,' she said hastily. 'Sparky just needs to recover and take it easy.'

'What do you mean "Take it easy?",' Ellen asked. 'What do dogs do that's hard?'

***

Sparky lay indolently on Chrissie's lap nibbling morsels of kosher chicken that Ellen had driven twenty-five minutes to purchase for dinner with her mother-in-law, Anne, who had not attended synagogue for eight years. Ellen, who was raised Catholic, suspected that these affectations in her mother-in-law, who dined several times a week in non-kosher restaurants, were retribution for naming her only granddaughter Christina.

Chrissie picked at the chicken breast; she did not eat meat with bones or in the presence of the carcass from which it came. Ground meat and sausages were fine, but she did not want any reminders of former corporeality.

'Don't feed the dog from the table,' Ellen said.

'Sparky likes it,' Chrissie said. 'I'm sure it's good for her.'

'Poor thing. You're nursing her back to health,' Anne said.

'*Pobre cita*,' Ellen lisped in mock sympathy. Ellen's older brothers had said this to her when she pleaded with their mother that she was too exhausted to do her chores.

'She barely eats anything now. I think she's depressed,' Chrissie said. 'From her ordeal,' she added with flourish. Chrissie, who – like Tom – did little to help around the house, dropped pieces of chicken on the floor.

Anne turned to Ellen. 'Are you feeding her now? Since her dog food is gluten-free, you can't claim that's a problem.'

Ellen, her face flushed, was about to speak before David cut in. 'Ellen took her to the vet. Otherwise, Sparky would have died.' To fill the void, he asked Chrissie to pass some apple cake. Chrissie passed it over Ellen's plate.

'Sorry Mom,' Chrissie said as a cake crumb fell into Ellen's bowl. Even though Ellen had told Anne not to bother to bring anything – whatever she brought would most certainly contain gluten as her mother-in-law felt that gluten-free food was only for the neurotic or eating-disordered – Anne persisted because 'Chrissie and Tom love my apple cake.'

Ellen pushed away her barely touched bowl of rice pudding. She would not be able to eat it now unless she served herself another portion in a new bowl.

Ellen watched the dog shuffle slowly along the floor to where Anne sat holding out a small piece of cake. 'I think there's something wrong with its hind legs,' Ellen said. 'It's moving them like they're a burden. Like they're not a part of its body. Look.'

'She's still recovering,' Anne said. 'She knows what's good. She's moving toward the cake.' The dog licked the cake off Anne's hand.

'I don't think it should be eating that.' Ellen looked on in disgust as Anne used the hand the dog licked to break off another piece of cake and pop it into her mouth.

The next day, when the dog soaked its bed with urine and refused to move, Ellen took it to the vet's again. The poisoning had sent the dog's adrenal glands on a kamikaze mission. 'Addison's disease is not that uncommon in dogs,' the vet said.

'Dogs get autoimmune diseases?'

'Sure. Sparky will need to take daily medication.'

'Will that help its legs?'

'Maybe.'

After a few weeks, Ellen was the only one remembering to give the dog its pills at the appropriate intervals. The children complained that it smelled and was boring; they rarely played with or cared for it. The dog alternated between not being able to go and wetting itself. It still couldn't lift its hind legs up very far. Ellen let the dog out in the backyard because walking was still too taxing for it, and she could hose it down afterwards.

Ellen moved the dog basket to the laundry room because of the odor. Whenever she swapped the old, urine-sodden towels for fresh ones, the dog looked at her gratefully before resting its head in its paws.

It was pathetic, Ellen thought.

***

Ellen's announcement that she was taking the dog for a walk did not seem odd to David and the kids who were absorbed in an episode of *Lost in Space*. The dog moved slowly, resting every half block, panting and exhausted. When Ellen tugged the leash, the dog picked itself up gingerly and walked with a staggering, crablike gait. Although Ellen slowed her pace to accommodate the dog, she felt a bit dizzy and wondered if her illness was now causing ataxia. She groped for the bag in her purse; had she forgotten it?

As they inched toward the park, jumbled thoughts ran through her foggy brain. *People didn't understand. At worst, they got the flu, a week's rest. A life spent in bed was no life at all.*

It could barely do anything anymore. Like some sick, old dog. I'll be doing it a favor...

This is what I'll tell them: Maybe Sparky ate some more moldy bread in the park, and it made her sick again... Or maybe the medicine wasn't really working. It didn't help with her legs, after all... She was already very sick. Maybe we didn't know how sick...

Ellen stopped for a moment. *No one would do an autopsy on a dog, would they?*

Once they entered the park, Ellen stuck her hand into her purse again, to remind herself of why they were there. She fingered the plastic bag containing the dog treats dusted with rat poison.

They walked past an elderly man sitting on a bench. His hand rested lightly atop his cane as if it were a rifle, ready to draw. While they passed down the path to the duck pond, his gaze tracked them like a target.

As they approached the pond, gangly Brett Carlsson, who used to make pig noises whenever Tom got on the school bus, skated toward them.

'Check out the drunk dog,' Brett scoffed to his friend as they flamingoed by on their skateboards. The other kid said, 'It's kind of fat too.' Ellen could hear them laughing long in the distance. She wanted to yell: 'It's water retention. And she's too sick to exercise!'

FINE NOW

Propped against the pond's weeping willow, like someone was drying them for stuffing, were slices of bread so green they glowed gently in the darkening light. *What kind of careless person does that?* Ellen wondered. The light croaking of frogs reverberated an answer: idiots, idiots, idiots.

Ellen sat on an empty bench facing the pond. The dog treats inside the plastic bag resembled uncooked schnitzel. Her hand shook as she placed the bag on the bench, and a rivulet of sweat ran down her temple despite the cool breeze. The dog wagged its tail excitedly, rubbed its face against her leg and sat in anticipation of a reward. For the first time that day, it seemed alert, interested. Its dark, liquid eyes looked up at her in expectation of some token of affection, a reward. A reward for what? Ellen reflected that the walk there had been arduous for the dog, which did not whine.

The long grasses rustled, and in the faint light, Ellen could make out a heron standing alert on a stone platform at the edge of the pond. With its still concentration and long, erect neck, for a moment, Ellen mistook it for a statue.

A flash of wings, and the heron was in the water. A frog dangled from its beak, firmly clamped with limbs rigid in animal pain and terror. The heron shook its head a few times, and the unlucky frog disappeared. The heron's neck bulged as the frog passed through. The other frogs, in their ignorance and apathy, continued to croak as if nothing had happened.

It was not the first time Ellen had seen a heron eat a frog, but she felt that she needed to vomit. There was bitterness and grief stuck in her throat that she had spent her entire life trying to clear. She coughed several times, startling the heron, which flew off, its neck curved in a smooth, elegant S. Ellen stared at the stone platform, empty except for a warped and gnarled piece of driftwood.

The dog had not witnessed the heron's casual brutality. It faced Ellen, waiting patiently for its treat. Ellen shivered; the park had grown ugly and cold. She stood up and put the bag into a trash can a few yards away. When she returned, the dog looked forlorn but did not whimper in disappointment. She patted its head. 'Let's go, Sparky.'

Tom peered into the picnic basket in the back seat. 'Rice crackers,' he said with distaste. 'What happened to the pretzels?'

'I've gotten rid of all the gluten.'

Tom scowled and slammed the door hard, his belly quivering from the effort.

Ellen walked past Tom and placed Sparky gently in the dog carrier in the back of the SUV, pushing aside a skateboard. Scratching behind Sparky's ears, Ellen said, '*Pobre cita*,' then stood aside as David loaded the fishing tackle and shut the hatch.

When they got to the lake, Ellen found that she couldn't face the boat or the sailing club's annual picnic on Apple Island. All those oblivious people. What would she miss, really?

'Are you sure you don't want to go?' David said as he boarded the boat. 'I should try to catch the wind.'

'Yes, we'll be just fine.' The castaways watched the boat sail away. Ellen waved back at Chrissie, and Sparky barked a few times.

Ellen thought that they would walk a little along the lake, but she could see that the dog was already making a strenuous effort to keep up. As they strolled back to the car, Sparky's crablike walk had the elements of a funny little dance. Ellen removed the skateboard from the trunk of the car and placed Sparky on it.

Pulling the dog along, Ellen smiled at Sparky standing erect and sturdy on the rolling skateboard, like a figurehead on the prow of a ship. Sparky barked excitedly, perhaps remembering the times, not long ago after all, when she ran so fast through the park, carefree.

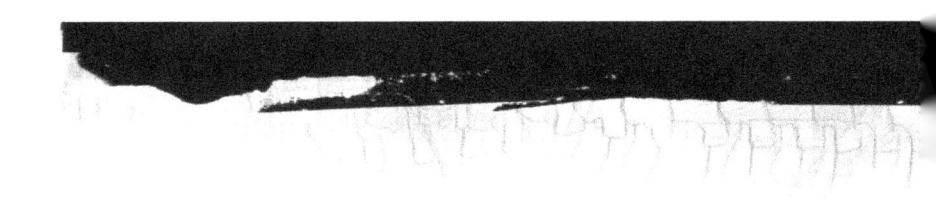

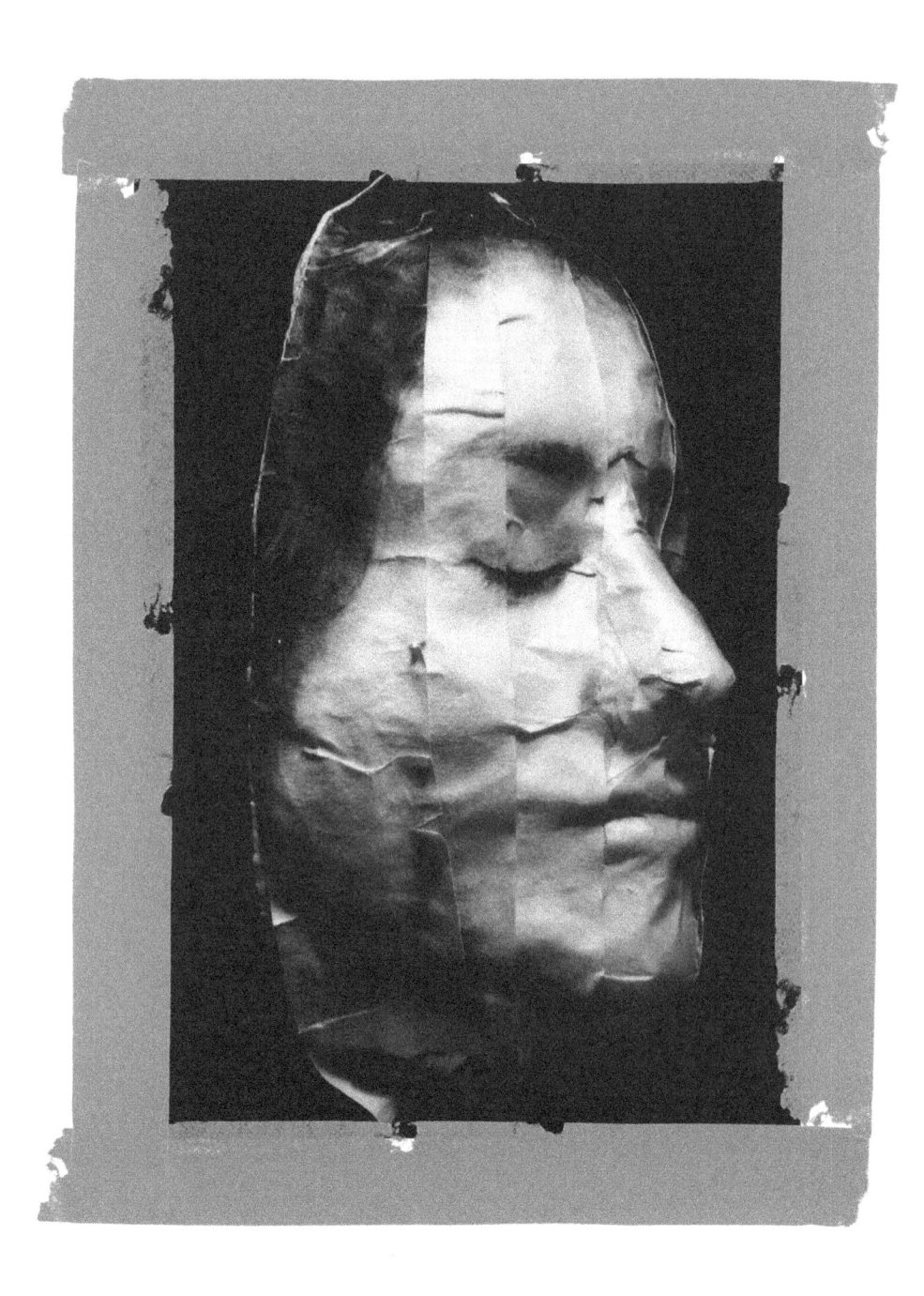

CARING FOR THE ASTILBES

by Shirley Muir

It was after his photograph appeared in the local newspaper, holding aloft the squash players' trophy, that we got the diagnosis. Standing in a hospital corridor, uniformed nurses and doctors jostling past, visiting relatives bumping against us, the consultant flicked through the thin pile of notes in his hand and said, 'I'm sorry, but it's malignant.'

***

Friends and family didn't ask, 'Is he going to die?' or 'Will he be all right?' They grimaced, made comments like, 'Oh god, sorry to hear that,' or 'It's amazing what they can do nowadays.'

We prepared in our heads a script of optimistic phrases like, 'I'm sure he'll be fine' or 'They're going to start treatment right away.' I trotted them out with contrived confidence. Jamie wasn't able to contrive any confidence.

Sipping cups of tea out of those china cups with a little cottage scene on them after the hundred-mile drive to my parents, we told my mother. I don't remember what she said but it included hugs and tissues and it was just right. My father was different. Shocked speechless that a fit, thirty-year-old sportsman would succumb to cancer, he had to sit down with a box of tissues to recover his composure. He wouldn't have held onto the little china cup or its saucer had he been clutching one.

On the way back home a couple of days later Jamie pulled into a layby on the wooded section of the major road half an hour short of Edinburgh. He turned off the engine and faced straight ahead, gripping the steering wheel 'til his knuckles were white. The sun shone on the little drips as they streamed down his face and fell onto his pale blue shirt, making dark patches.

'I don't think I can do this,' he said. We hugged and clutched one another, then we sobbed until we were both very wet. We had to open the car windows to demist them.

We made a plan to save us having to repeat to others the horror of receiving the diagnosis in that crowded hospital passageway. Another trip by car to inform his parents was next but after that we would take it slowly, asking both sets of parents to tell aunts and uncles and siblings and family friends and acquaintances. And we promised to keep the parents informed of progress over the coming months.

Although responses from friends and family as we told them were well-meant, many felt banal. But friends and family have to get you through this, whatever their first response. I have been very banal myself and been forgiven for it.

'Is there anything you need?' my friend Susan asked after she'd stroked my hands and kissed my fingers.

'Yes,' I thought. 'I want this all to be a bad dream. I want it to go away so we can wake up.'

I said, 'He loves crosswords. Perhaps a crossword book. Thank you.'

I didn't say, 'Please don't give him novels about people with cancer,' as Aunty Jill did, innocently. Bless her. Or American books on how you can cure cancer without medical treatment.

I didn't say, 'Please don't give him stories about miracles or about taking control of your own life. Don't tell us that having a positive outlook will enable him to survive.'

Because that really means if he dies then it will be his own fault.

***

I visit the isolation ward and pull on latex gloves and tie the obligatory face mask and slip on the elasticated nylon hair cap. After an astonishing twenty-year cancer conflict with a battalion of chemotherapy drugs and newly-discovered monoclonal antibody therapy, the disease is still growing and spreading inside Jamie's battered body. Fewer medical options remain to us. This is my first visit since he was bombarded by the massive dose of chemotherapy, which precedes the gruelling, life-threatening-life-saving stem cell transplant.

'What actually happens,' the no-nonsense consultant said, 'is they almost kill you then they bring you back from the brink.' Newly infused with clean, life-giving blood cells.

But this ammunition is composed of his own blood cells. They 'cleaned them up' a bit. He has six siblings and not one of them was a suitable match. Close sibling matches, not exact matches, give the best result, the consultant said.

Fighting his leukaemia means that Jamie's own immune system is virtually wiped out. It might let him down badly. That's a euphemism. I know he could die from a sore throat or a cut finger.

So here we are in the sterile unit where he needs to live for an unknown period of time. Armies of new stem cells storm into his bloodstream from a small plastic packet above his head through a thin transparent plastic line. I watch them streaming to the rescue, although they look to me just like ordinary flowing blood. I encourage them in whispers to flood through his veins, seek their new home in his bones, conquer the enemy lymphocytes and colonise his deliberately depleted bone marrow.

'I've brought you a newspaper,' I say in a muffled voice through the fabric of the face mask.

The ghostly figure on a white sheet in a sterile white room doesn't move. Weak as a kitten, his face as waxen as the candles I have been lighting for him in every church I pass, his attachment to life is as fine as a silken thread. I pray that the mask will disguise my terror and conceal my own pallid face.

From the surreal blandness of the bed in the isolation room his azure eyes flicker open.

That blue gaze pierces my soul. It mirrors the colour of the Mediterranean where we snorkelled hand in hand through blizzards of silvery, pink, and yellow fish. We revelled in the warmth of the sea caressing our bodies and the passing crowds of oblivious, rainbow-hued creatures that shone against the golden backdrop of the sandy seabed. A bold fish might stroke a leg or nudge an arm, creating a tickling sensation or a frisson of fear.

It was only last year.

Through dry, cracked lips he croaks, 'Hello.'

Then he says, 'This is like that scene in *2001: A Space Odyssey* where the astronaut is lying in a white bed in a white room, near the end of the film. Remember?' I nod. It's his favourite film and the early scene with the fanfare of Strauss's *Also Sprach Zarathustra* is one of the most-played vinyl LPs on our home stereo system.

I slide onto the hard, upright hospital chair that someone has recently sterilised. Every item in his room is germ-free. My focus moves to the plastic line that snakes from today's bag of colourless liquid on a hanger above his head down into a plastic valve they have installed on the right of his chest. It's an antibiotic this time, to protect him until his immune system can start again to do its job.

'I watered the Astilbes,' I say. 'They are doing well in this nice warm weather.'

He planted six Astilbes, three white and three red, around the edge of the lawn, as dusk fell on the night before his hospital admission. He carefully selected Astilbes – a colourful option for our shady back garden.

'And I brought you the newspaper with the crossword.' It surprises me that they don't seem to need to sterilise newspapers.

'Sorry,' he murmurs, opening his eyes after an unintended snooze, 'I can't concentrate. I can't even read the headlines, but do leave the newspaper. You never know...'

His lids fall heavily and consciousness peters out. For a while I watch over him. If I am there nothing bad can happen. Time passes without me noticing or caring.

A week slips by with daily visits at any hour that suits me; all the days are identical for me except Sunday when there's less traffic rumbling by the living room windows where I drink coffee before I walk to the hospital along the arterial road that hums with traffic day and night. Where can they all be going? Why don't they know how sad I am? I have to steer my thoughts to focus on that white room, and not consider the bliss of stepping in front of a juggernaut to put an end to this horror.

Each night, as dusk descends, I converse with the new tenants of our garden. I sluice cool water onto their roots.

'Have a little drink, Astilbes,' I say. 'Grow strong and healthy.' In the gloom I tell them how he was today. How he asks after them every day. And he promises to see them soon.

His face lights up each time I appear beside him in the glare of the white room. My heart stands still in response. These times together are uneventful, but prized like jewels. I collect the jewels in a special box of memory, one after another. I wonder how it will end. How many jewels I will have.

'I did twelve across,' he whispers one day, in obvious pain from the havoc-wreaking mouth ulcers that inhibit eating or speaking. It's the same crossword from the early days of the transplant. A few short weeks ago. The newspaper has become dog-eared but he won't let them bin it. Perhaps they've microwaved it.

'I'm sorry, I have no conversation, not in here with no connection to the outside world. I might never see it again anyway.'

'I'm not interested in the Middle East or the price of milk or the train strike.' I smile. 'Just you.'

He used to tell me to take note of current affairs, to be aware of the world around me, to care about the actions of statesmen, of politicians, of presidents. I tried. I learned about dictators ruling the nations of the Middle East, about countries applying desperately for acceptance into the European Union. I read about the multi-party parliamentary system that operates in the UK and why the people of Scotland wanted independence.

Next time I visit, the ulcers have abated slightly. He sips a spoonful of warm lentil soup.

'Three more clues yesterday,' he says, 'in an hour.' His breathing is laboured, he wheezes, a lung infection lurking beneath the words he utters.

'I got Sisyphus, the over-proud king who had to push a large boulder uphill forever as a punishment. Then I fell asleep.' His body is suddenly wracked by an alarming fit of coughing. I wait, tense, patient. I pray. I want to cover my ears but it would be crass.

And then, looking up at me, he quietens and says, 'Did you water...?' I nod.

'I did, and the flowers are out now, so pretty. The red ones at the left side of the garden are taller than the white ones on the right.'

'There used to be a compost heap there, that's why,' he pants, the effort straining his lungs again. He closes his eyes and the wheezing grows loud and terrifying.

He remembers about the compost heap and our hopes for Galapagos-dimension progress from the geraniums and fuchsias and begonias we planted on it last year. We had discovered extraordinarily fertile soil on the left side of the garden and the neighbour had mentioned it had been the location for the previous owner's garden rubbish that became a mountainous compost heap.

***

Another week flies past. His damaged and cracked lips heal enough to allow a small piece of soft bread between sips of mushroom soup. Then the soup reminds him that the lining of his mouth is still scored with deep, stinging ulcers. Like drinking acid, he says.

My heart clenches in pain as the blue eyes hold my gaze.

'It rained torrentially in the night on Sunday,' I tell him, 'so your Astilbes didn't need water from my watering can. They've got big flowers now. Six inches high, each bloom.'

'I heard the rain splashing off these windows,' he says, and sinks back into the pillows. 'They prefer rain water, you know, better than tap water. What's the chemical in tap water?'

'Chlorine,' I say.

He nods. I mop a dribble of mushroom soup from his chin.

'I've done nearly half of that crossword,' he says, his voice dazed and uncertain.

I nod again.

'You mustn't do any, though,' he mutters with surprising energy. 'It's a barometer for my recovery.'

My heart contracts with desperate love. I can feel my eyes prickle but fight back the tears.

But he's drifted away from me.

***

Two weeks later I'm startled to find him sitting on the side of the bed in his outdoor clothes. A white paper bag sealed with a pharmacist's label sits beside him. It bulges with boxes and packets of life-saving medication. Antibiotics, mouthwashes, painkillers, anti-sickness tablets, steroids, gut adjusters.

He hands me the crinkled page with the old crossword.

'Fifteen down,' he says. A weak smile cracks his dry, white lips. 'Something completed.'

'Finished,' I read.

I grin. I know that we'll have a long haul from here. Together. But that important part is finished for now.

And I realise that the banality of 'It's amazing what they can do nowadays' isn't banal at all. During the cancer conflict we have lived over the past twenty years he's benefitted from monoclonal antibodies, a specialised radiotherapy treatment for his eye, and now this revolutionary stem cell procedure – and probably a handful of relatively ordinary drugs that have extended his grip on life.

I stuff the bulging bag of life-saving potions into his holdall along with the pyjamas, crossword book and unread, old newspapers. 'No, I don't need a wheelchair,' he grumps, 'I'm not incapable, you know.'

Leaning heavily on my arm and walking like a fragile, sick man, he holds my left hand in his. Such limited strength is in that hand today. Not the power of a trophy-winning squash player smashing the hundred-mile-an-hour squash ball against the wall at the peak of human fitness.

He raises my hand and brushes it with his scratchy, damaged lips. Tears trickle unexpectedly down my face.

Together we shuffle towards the EXIT sign at the end of the corridor.

'I never expected to walk under this sign again,' he gasps, and halts for a moment, drained by the physical effort of the very short stroll. I stifle my desire to call for that wheelchair.

'Well, the Astilbes are expecting you.'

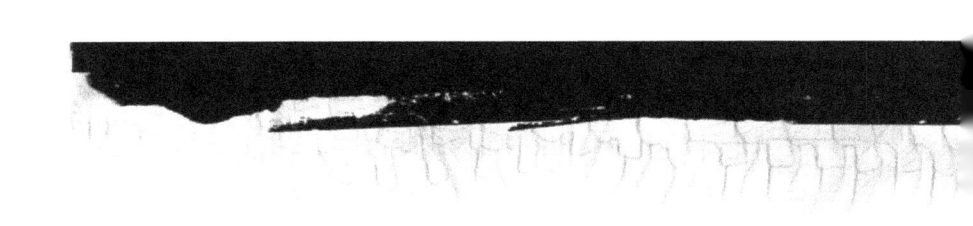

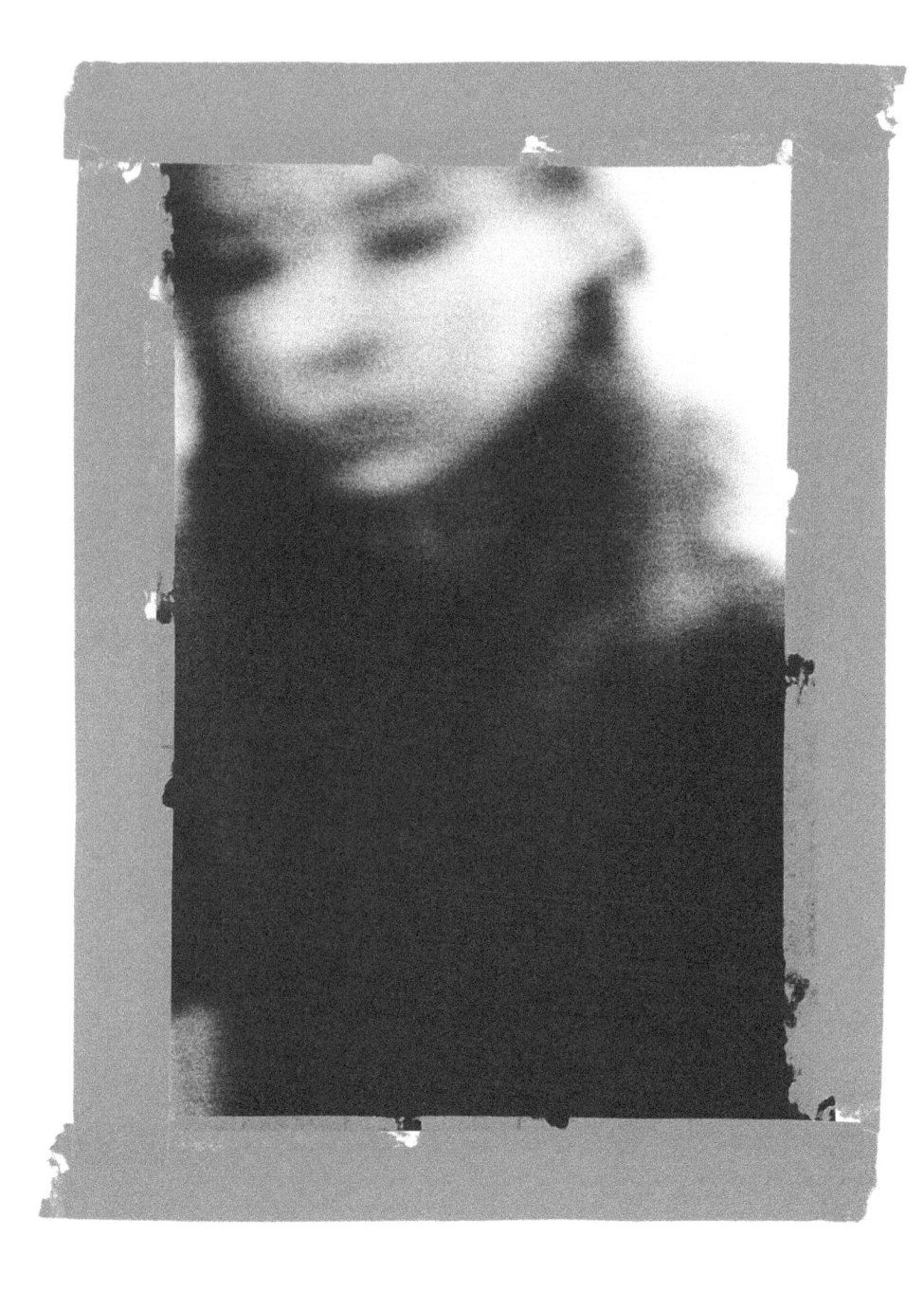

HIDDEN IN PLAIN SIGHT

by Bea Mulder, aged 12 at time of writing

~~Normalness~~

I always wanted to be normal.
Normal life.
Normal girl.
Normal friends.

But I gave up on my dreams of normality,
The day It happened.

And this is It.

Chapter 1

Water-logged clouds heave their sodden selves miserably across the sky, threatening to let loose and drench the land beneath them.
   I awake drowsily and heave myself out of bed. Dragging my feet across my cramped bedroom. Stumbling blindly to the mirror. As I rub my eyes, my brain does not at first fully register what I am seeing. Or rather what I am not seeing…

A gasp escapes my lips. I feel my body freeze. I am a statue of cement, frozen in shock. Terrified by the sight that has greeted me in my awakening hours, I stumble backwards.

There is no reflection.

There is no me.

A million thoughts sound in my head. Yet I don't move. I'm so shocked I can only stay silent. I bring my hands up right before my face but I'm still staring blankly at the empty mirror. I keep my eyes open and press my trembling fingers into them. I rub violently and wince as they begin to water. However, my view of the mirror is just as clear and steady as usual. Then it hits me, not only my reflection has vanished but so have I.

Numbly I reach out what I feel to be a shaking hand. My clammy fingers make contact with the undisturbed glass and complex fingerprints appear on the lustrous surface. My analytical mind tells me that what I'm seeing is simply not possible, but it is happening, right before my eyes. I stare, entranced, at the interconnecting lines until they swim under my gaze. This is part of me and as I feel myself begin to slip away, I want to keep them in my sight forever.

But they disappear, and I am left with an empty hand and empty hope. A beat passes. Hysterical panic consumes me next and I'm crying and screaming and mumbling all at the same time. Confusion and delusion devour me as I drop to the floor hopelessly. A sodden pile of nothingness.

I am nothing.

I no longer matter.

Nothing I ever do will make any kind of difference and I will never know why.

What is the point of living anymore?

Chapter 2

Finally, I manage to regain my feet and shuffle jerkily to the mirror once more. Its empty surface still makes me gasp but I clench my fists, grit my teeth and walk out of the door.

It's Friday so Mum is out and won't be back 'til later, I have the whole house to myself until then. Meanwhile I try not to think about how I'm going to explain to her what has happened to me.

I don't know how she is going to react when she realises how this will tear our relationship apart. Mum's always been so incredibly supportive and I don't think our bond could become any closer. When she hears that I'm leaving home, I don't want to see her face. I don't want to see the tracks of her tears.

It will be better this way. That's what I tell myself.
I will be happier this way. That's what I tell myself.
No one will miss me. That's what I tell myself.

This is the right choice. The pain of being here but not being *fully* present would be too much to bear for me and Mum.

As if in a trance, I tiptoe slowly down the stairs. I take small mechanical steps, still in shock. I am aiming to be packed by the time Mum arrives home. A quick goodbye. That's what it must be. If not, I know I will lose my resolve and with it my chance.

I *need* to be strong, for her and for me.
I *must* be strong.

Once downstairs I creep into the kitchen. The blinds are still drawn so Mum must have left for work in a rush. Being a teaching assistant means you can't afford to be late. It comes as quick as that and I find myself bent over in emotional pain.

***

I was eight. We were lying on the sofa, the film had finished. The credits were rolling on and the tinny music accompanied them. Mum was absentmindedly stroking my cheek. I was deep in thought, concentrating hard on a dancing ember in the dying fire.

'Mum?' I ask sleepily.
'Yes darling?'
'Do you love the children you teach as much as you love me?'
There's a short silence and I hold my breath.

'No darling, of course not. I look after them, and I care for them, and I'm fond of them, but I have a special love for you. You are my daughter, and no mother could love their daughter as much as I love you.'
I heave a sigh of relief and persist,
'But Mum... Doesn't everyone Mum say that to their daughter?'
I can feel her smile.
'You are a wise girl Leah, and yes, perhaps some other mothers say that to their children too but know this: I. Love. You. And that is all that matters.'
'Okay,' I grin as I drop off to sleep.
I feel her chest rise and fall beneath me and I cuddle up close to her. I don't think I have ever felt safer in my life.

***

The memory brings a fresh wave of despair. My eyes sting but I squint hard and somehow manage to choke back the tears. Maybe this isn't a good idea. Maybe this is dangerous. Maybe I should stay.
I gulp, open my eyes, stand up straight and push the nagging doubt away as I carry on with the task in hand.

Chapter 3

Six slices of bread; ham; cheese; leftover jam; two chicken drumsticks; a small bottle of milk; three breadsticks and two chocolate bars.
These are my rations after half an hour of self-debate. I pack only the essentials; things Mum probably won't notice are missing. It was tempting to add in a slice of banana cake to the mix but I decide against it.
Another two hours are left to prepare myself for the big leap. Carefully I load the food into a Sainsbury's carrier bag and leave it in position by the front door. I am then a whirlwind of organisation. By 3pm I have finished. A large backpack and the small food bag are waiting for me by the door. I still have half an hour before Mum arrives home. I bite my lip hard. I am surprised to find myself welcoming the fresh pain and do it again, and again. Each sharp nip sends a shooting

pain through my mouth and stops me from crumpling into a sobbing heap. I am left with a shredded lip and the metallic taste of blood in my mouth.

What am I going to do with my life?

For the remaining time, I glumly watch as the hands on the clock chase each other round its face. Then the doorbell rings.

She's back.

Mum sweeps in, like a muddled hurricane of chaos. A tsunami of brightly-coloured clothing and countless shopping bags. After re-arranging her eccentric self she finally looks up.

I gasp quietly, taken aback by how *alive* she looks.

I want to count each of her eyelashes. I want to trace the faint lines in her forehead with my finger, most of all, I just want to hold her.

Mum's eyes flit upwards, she doesn't know I'm watching her. She looks through me. I shiver and promise myself I will forget this eerie image. I don't want to remember my mum like this. Unseeing and unknowing.

Slowly she tilts her head from side to side, as if she can sense something is wrong. 'Leah?' she calls in the direction of the stairs. I don't know what I'm going to say, or how I'm going to say it, but somehow...

I speak.

'Hi Mum,' I say. I hold my breath as I wait for the reaction. Her head whirls towards the sound, wavy chocolate brown hair catching the air. Taking a deep breath she asks, 'Are you hiding?'

Our dining room is set out all in plain view. The table is high and the cupboards are full and pushed against the wall. There is no way I could be hiding in this room, and she knows it.

'No, Mum,' I answer quietly.

'Then where in heaven's name are you?'

I can tell she is trying to hide how very scared she is. 'At the table,' I reply bluntly. Mum blinks once, then twice. Her face breaks into a smile and creases appear at the corners of her eye. Soon she's bent double with laughter.

'Mum,' I whisper. No reply.

'Mum,' I say, a little louder this time. No reply.

'Mum!' I shout. She suddenly stands straight. The ghost of a smile that still remained on her face quickly vanishes. Heart-breaking worry registers on Mum's gentle face and I just want to get it over and done with as soon as possible.

'I'm here,' I speak shakily. Silence stretches between us. Heart hammering, I stand up. I watch her eyes track the chair as it pulls itself away from the table. Her mouth is hanging open, eyes wide, fists clenched. She's swaying ever so slightly, I want to go and help her. Steady her, but I know I can't.

'I'm sorry,' I whisper. Mum bursts into tears and stumbles blindly towards me, nearly knocking over two chairs. Instinctively I start towards her, arms outstretched, but then I pause and back away from this sudden outburst as I quickly consider my options.

Option 1 – Comfort her.

Option 2 – Leave.

I choose Option 2.

Chapter 4

The goodbye didn't go as I had hoped it would. I crept quietly across the kitchen – eyes squeezed tightly shut so that no stray tears would escape – picked up the bags and tiptoed cautiously to the door. I reached out a hand and twisted the handle. The door creaked, long and loud as if relishing in its destruction.

The last memories of my mum were scarred forever.

She barreled towards me. Her cheeks were tear-stained and swollen, her eyes searched blindly. She was moaning and muttering my name. I took a deep breath and walked out of the door.

When I think of my mum now, all I see in my mind is her face as I last saw it. Betrayed, hysterical, and heart-broken.

I don't see the many memories we shared. The cookie making. The lazy mornings in bed. The conversations. Or the cuddles.

All I see is her tortured face. Eyes wild with sadness. Shouting and screaming.

Being so unlike herself.
And I hate myself for it.

Chapter 5

Rubbish is strewn across the ground in careless heaps. Rats scurry from pile to pile seeking shelter. I hug my knees and rock back and forth, dreading my future in this new life. It's 4pm on a Thursday and six days have passed since I left home. It's amazing what that amount of time with no human contact can do to the soul. I am the shell of the girl I once was. Unwashed and unclean, with no hope.

The nights have been the worst. Curled into a tight ball, eyes squeezed shut, with only sheets of newspaper between my body and the grimy ground. I always awaken alert yet bedraggled, ready to leap to my feet, grab my bags and run. I will have to start scavenging soon.

If I wasn't invisible I can imagine what a wreck I would look. Wide sunken eyes, a tangled mess of unruly hair, dust-stained skin.

Voices drift my way. A small smile takes over my face, I can't help it. Freya. Freya, my friend.

Her velvety auburn hair bobs into view, silky locks catching the autumn breeze. Her carefree smile is contagious. Freya was there for me at a time where no body else was. In our early primary school years we didn't really know each other. An occasional smile or a subtle nod was the only communication that really passed between us. Throughout Year 4 it became apparent that we were more similar than we had thought. Two outcasts, reaching out to each other. However it was she who took the first steps.

***

Art. My favourite lesson. I sit in the corner of the classroom by myself – as usual. I don't really mind, it gives me lots of time to dream. The creation of the world. Human behavior. Evolution... I have plenty to think about.

My art supplies are in front of me; stationery to the left, pencils in the middle and spare paper to the right.

I notice a few critical glances shot my way but I don't understand. It makes sense to have everything organised. I look down, my hands itching to draw. Finally, Mrs Abbott finishes droning on and lets us work. I start off by sketching. The pencil brushes against the paper, bruising its surface. Lightly, I sketch the outline. The outline of what, I have yet to find out. Gradually fur begins to grow and my wolf evolves. After thirty-five minutes she is staring back at me. Teeth bared. Hackles raised. Eyes, piercing through mine, making me shiver.

I put my pencil down, lean back in my chair and stretch as I admire my artwork. Breath. Breath on the back of my neck. For a fleeting moment I think that my wolf has come to life and is standing behind me. I whirl around and I am met with much, much worse than a wolf. Mrs Abbott's sickly smiling face greets me. 'What's this you've drawn, Leah?' she asks stickily.

'It's a wolf,' I say, wondering how she hadn't noticed this.

A look of annoyance crosses her face and is quickly replaced with a painted smile that reveals too many of her teeth.

'Leah,' she grimaces, 'is this,' she indicates a wrinkled finger towards my snarling wolf, 'what I told you to draw?'

I feel furious, my anger bubbles within like lava in a volcano. I long to let it out, to let it burn her, to let it hurt her. But I am silent.

She smirks. Suddenly her face is right down close to mine, only a few centimeters between us. Her sticky stench is overwhelming. 'I advise,' she spits, words plucked and sharp, 'you dispose of this immediately.'

Then she sweeps away, as though nothing has happened. Hands shaking, I reach out for the drawing, ready to put it in my bag. Another hand suddenly grips my wrist and Jack Konwey's eyes meet mine. He smiles and twists my arm back. Held there, unable to move, I watch helplessly as my wolf is defaced. His friends laugh as they draw crude moustaches and ugly doodles with felt-tips on her beautiful face. 'Stop,' I whisper.

'What was that?' Jack mocks.

'Stop,' I repeat, a fraction louder.

'No,' he sneers, 'if you're not going to bin it, then I will. Bring it here,' he calls to the others. They wave it tauntingly in my face, Jack grabs it. He's *about to rip it, I close my eyes, but the tearing sound doesn't come.*

I open my eyes to see a girl with red hair come charging towards Jack, she knocks him over and I hear the thump of his head against the floor.

Events turn fast. Eyes. Thirty pairs of staring eyes trained on me and Freya. There's a brief moment of silence. She looks at me, I smile gingerly and she smiles back; warmly but with a definite hint of danger. She let her lava loose, she let it burn. Her hair is a halo of fire blazing bright in defiance, she isn't sorry for what she's done. She's proud. 'Thank you,' I manage to mouth just before Freya is dragged away by Mrs Abbott. The wolf has pounced.

***

I finally had someone – besides Mum – to share my ideas and thoughts with. We made each other strong and somehow survived the transition from primary to secondary school. I wonder where she thinks I am as she hasn't seen me since Thursday... I decide to follow her.

Not wanting to be heard, I sit up and peel the newspaper off my palm. After gaining my feet and stretching my stiff legs, I creep out of the foul alley. In the park across the road sits Freya, laughing at something someone has said. I run across the road and look up at Freya, excitement bubbling. Then my smile vanishes. I stumble backwards. The grass scratches my skin. The sun retreats and a chill climbs up my arms. In front of me is a scene that simply isn't possible. Freya, *my* friend sitting next to *her*.

***

We're halfway through Year 5 when Nikki joins the school. She flounces into the classroom like she owns the place. All eyes are on her. No-one has ever seen anyone like her. Short skirt, ornate handbag and a face plastered in make-up. Freya and I exchange sceptical glances, who is this? Nikki's striking hazel eyes meet mine, I gulp and try to look somewhere else. She has a strange aura around her, and I can feel her sizing me up.

***

Nikki's dazzling smile and pathetic giggle make me feel sick. Freya's laughing too but it sounds alien to my ears. This isn't the girl I once knew so well. Her laugh sounds taunting, and I edge nearer. Freya's lips are pink and her eyebrows are drawn on, what has Nikki done to my friend?

I sit down on the grass and listen to their conversation. It's gossip. Over the next half an hour I learn many pointless things such as who's going out with who, who tripped over in the canteen and which eyeliner is the best.

Finally their chat comes to an end and they stand up. 'See you tomorrow,' Freya calls to Nikki. Dismayed, I sit and watch as my friend walks off into the distance, her skirt raised and a new handbag swinging around her wrist.

Chapter 6

Stunned, I trail back to the alley. Thoughts squirm around in my head. It doesn't make sense. Arms around my knees I watch the sun retreat behind the horizon. Tears trickle down my cheeks as I quietly cry myself to sleep.

I awake to the sound of heavy breathing and the rustle of a plastic bag. It takes a moment to focus in the autumn mist. The dustbin man's cold breath is a cloud of fog, floating into nothingness. Shivering, I watch his gloved hands fumble with the bin lining as he tries to loosen it. Finally, he detaches it and hauls the bag to the truck. Then he climbs into the passenger seat and is gone.

Judging by the dim light, it is around 6:30am. Friday. I yawn as I rearrange my belongings but then something catches my eye: a pencil. I scramble to remove the newspaper that covers it. Hidden underneath is buried treasure: my art materials. I'd forgotten that I packed them. Paper, pencils, rubber, sharpener – just the basics but I still stare in wonder at the rubies and diamonds I have found. I draw – it helps me think. Slowly but surely a plan begins to form and my hope is reignited. A garden grows on my paper, flowers bloom as I sketch and vines climb out of my pencil. I laugh and at last feel happiness. For once in a long time I begin to think that maybe, just maybe, I might have a chance in this life.

An hour passes and I become immersed in my artwork. I can almost hear the bees buzzing. I can almost feel the gentle spring breeze that rustles through the trees. When I am finished I hide my treasure safely under my jacket and stand up. Repeating yesterday, I cross the road and settle myself comfortably on a bench. Ten minutes roll by and I start to worry. What if Freya doesn't turn up? Relief washes over me when I eventually hear her voice. However I bristle when I hear Nikki's chime alongside Freya's. As they pass by – giggling like maniacs – I slip off my bench and join them, careful to keep in step to prevent them noticing the extra tapping of my feet. More people are awake now and the gentle hum of voices increases. I'm relieved, it means I am less likely to be heard.

When the school comes into sight I see Mum at the school gates.

All my emotions magnify. I'm instantly immersed under the surface of sadness. Her face. Her pain, reflecting my own. She looks older than before and her eyes sag into her face. Fists clenched as she walks. I long to run to her, to tell I am here, but I can't – it would only increase her longing. Frightened by how much she has changed, I dart ahead and join a small group of teens who are hanging around outside the gates – I'm just within earshot of her. 'Have you seen my daughter?' she asks anyone she can. Desperation seeps into her begging voice and it is painful to listen to. Most people walk on, stone faced and seemingly oblivious, but I know they can hear her. They are too wrapped up in their own problems to worry about one missing child. Some offer looks of sympathy but that won't bring me back. Nothing will.

Freya and Nikki have caught up now, and out of the corner of my eye I spot Freya falter. She stops and Nikki rolls her eyes. 'Come *on* Freya, we're going to be late.'

'Hang on...' Freya murmurs, a strange look in her eyes. She's spotted Mum. Mum spots her.

'Freya!' Mum exclaims, her last spark of hope working its way to the surface. 'Have you seen Leah?' she pleads. I expect she already knows the answer but she doesn't want to have to accept the truth. The truth that I am gone. Is she blaming herself? Does she think she's gone mad? Life will never be the same for her again. Freya's face crumples. 'She isn't with you?' comes the stricken reply.

Without saying a word, Mum stoops to pick up her bag and walks slowly away. Tears roll down my cheeks as I watch her broken figure fade and she disappears from sight.

Chapter 7

'Come *on*.' Nikki's harsh command makes me jump and I snap back to reality.

'But Nikki... Leah... She's missing,' Freya's muttering uncomfortably.

'Yeah, so what?' Nikki scoffs, 'You don't still want to be friends with her do you? She was such a loser.'

'No, but... she's missing...' Sheepish words – what has happened to the passionate girl I once knew? What has happened to Freya's flame?

'Then come *on*, we're going to be late!' Nikki is relentless and finally Freya reluctantly lets her drag her through the gates. Just before they enter the crowd Freya looks over her shoulder, a look of unease on her face. For a moment it seems like she is staring right at me, I gaze back and raise a timid hand in an unsaid farewell. Then Nikki tugs her sleeve and the moment is broken. At least I got to say goodbye.

Turning away from the school. Walking back the way I came. Watching, listening. Numb, removed. I don't belong here. The hum of voices sound alien to my ears. The grass seems too green and the trees too tall. Dazed and detached, I wander through the streets until I reach the alley. My cold fingers grasp at the few belongings that I have left. I slip the backpack on, it's worryingly lighter than I remember, and begin my journey. I wander through the streets silently observing and collecting memories, paying attention to every detail. A toddler screaming at his mum, an elderly lady returning from the shops, a man bending down to tie his shoelaces. My mind is a camera; my eyes are the shutter; my memories are the photos. Each scene overlaps like blueprints in a dark room; I store them all up on a shelf and promise myself that I will look through them later.

Not wanting to miss anything, I retrace my steps again and again, breathing in the familiarity that is my home. Conflicting emotions churn within me; joy at the sight of all that I've been lucky enough to endure, and sorrow at the thought of all that I am leaving behind. An hour passes. Then two, then three, and I lose myself in the beautiful chaos.

Eventually, at one o'clock, I manage to tear myself away. My destination is only a short way down the road, but I try to take as long as possible, savouring every moment here. The train station blurs into view and a thrill stirs within me. My pace quickens and excitement overrides terror. Noise from the village slowly quietens and then all is silent.

I sit upon a bench on the deserted platform, and my legs swing rhythmically as I wait in anticipation for the train.

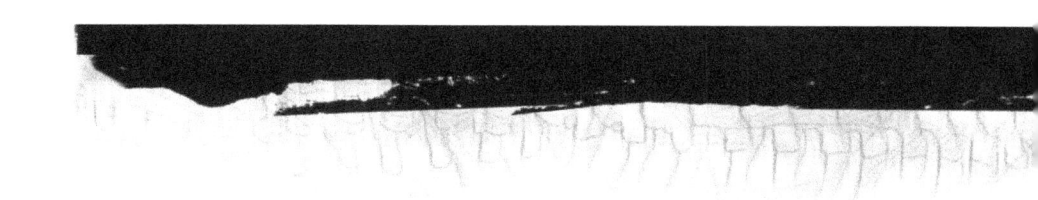

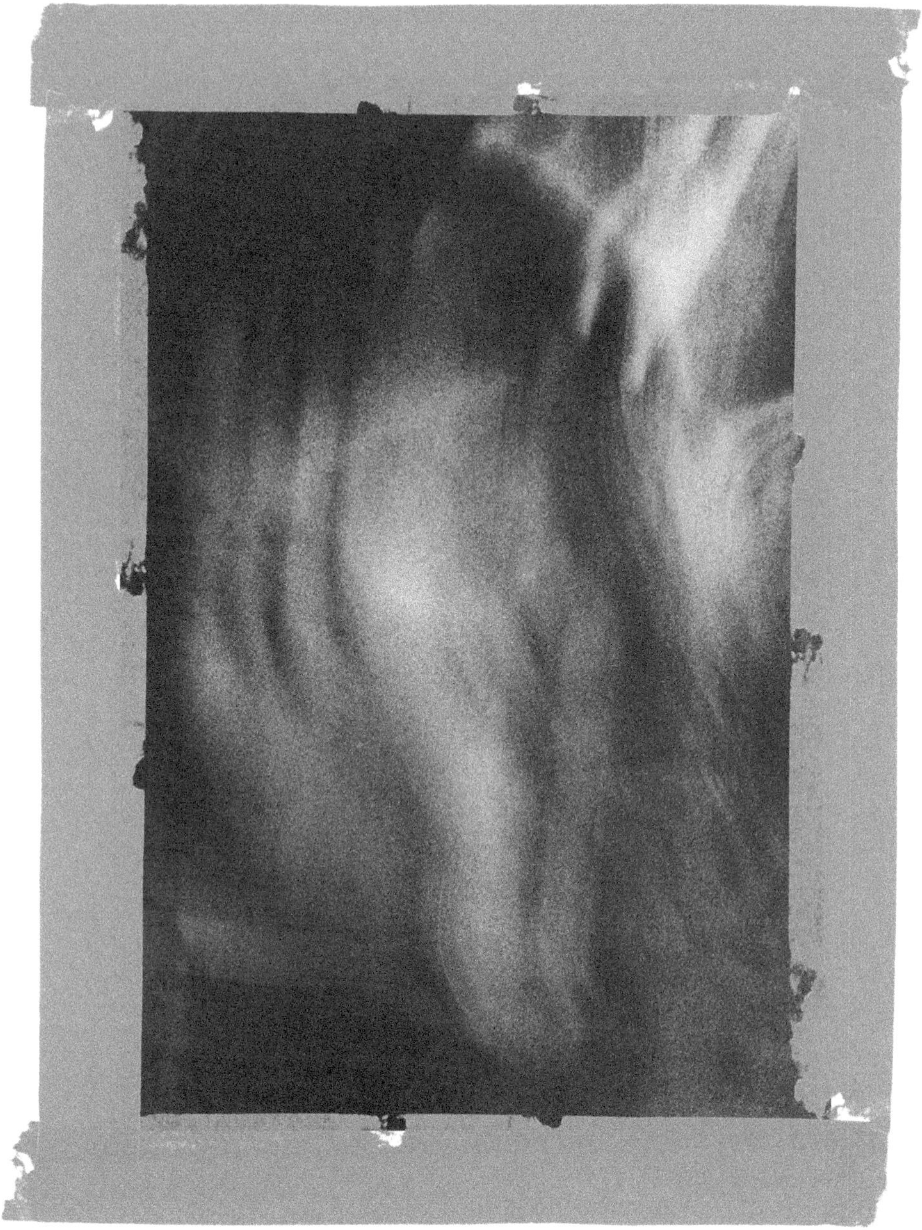

A NEW LEASE OF LIFE

by Neel Patel

As the assimilation party who had relayed the news observed our group, I was certain that several of them were casting glances in my direction. It could have been paranoia; I was jet-lagged, hungover, and disorientated from what I'd been informed was an undulation in the space-time continuum; a concept my sleep-deprived mind was struggling to absorb in the wake of the revelations that had greeted me upon landing.

I sympathised with our welcoming committee. How to optimally convey to a planeload of disgruntled and confused travellers from Tokyo that they had arrived twenty years into the future was beyond me: to be responsible for informing a pack of strangers that their parents had died, children had grown up, jobs were redundant, homes repossessed, spouses remarried... compared to all that, the space-time continuum part seemed almost inconsequential.

The murmur amongst my fellow passengers had risen to a panicked chatter as they repeated what they had heard to themselves in the vain hope that it would make sense. The eyes of the Homeland Security personnel widened in discomfort as they were subjected to a series of questions. As the cacophony in the basement room of San Francisco International Airport reached a crescendo, the door opened and several

JNS airline staff entered, carrying a stack of parcels. Their arrival was met with relief by the Homeland Security team, one of whom clapped his hands for attention.

'Ladies and gentlemen,' he began. 'If I may – my name is Jonathan Hoynes. I appreciate that this is an extremely challenging experience for you all and that you have many questions. Please be assured that we will do our best to help you adjust to this new reality. In the meantime...' he waved one of the parcels. 'Courtesy of JNS airlines, we have the following tablets, pre-loaded with orientation tutorials to help familiarise you with life in 2037.'

I marvelled at the effect that a brand new, shiny tablet could have on a person, even twenty years on. The group fell silent as the parcels were handed out. I opened mine and took out a featherweight black slate, which lit up as soon as I touched the screen to show a message offering me the option of priming it with my thumbprint.

'They're so thin!' exclaimed the man to my right, his earlier concerns seemingly forgotten as he blinked appreciatively at his new accessory.

'Indeed,' beamed Hoynes. 'The first graphene tablets were introduced about fifteen years ago. The tutorial can be found on the top right of the home screen.' His attention was averted briefly as he checked his watch, a look of gratitude appearing on his face. 'It appears that the first batch of friends and family have arrived to pick several of you up. We will call out the names of those who they've come to collect shortly. The remainder will be put up for the evening at the nearby Hyatt Regency, once again courtesy of our friends over at JNS.'

Forty-five minutes later I was sitting in an underground shuttle hurtling towards the Hyatt Regency. Unlike most of the others, I wasn't despondent about not having been collected by anyone. As far as I was concerned, there was no one in San Francisco who knew Howard DeMille from Northolt in the United Kingdom. I had been relatively quiet back at the airport. Whilst the other passengers had interrogated the Homeland Security team with constant questions about the brave new world we'd found ourselves in, I had sat back, slowly digesting my situation with an increasing sense of relief.

If this was 2037, then I didn't need to follow through.

This state of calm had probably been mistaken for shock by those around me. All throughout the flight, I had been struggling internally with the task that awaited me in San Francisco; the immensity of what I had to do... only for it all to fall apart upon landing, removing all my responsibilities and cares. There had only been Ryan I needed to think about and it was highly unlikely he would still be alive after all this time. Even if they had found a cure in the last generation, who but me would have cared enough to have sourced, researched, and paid for it? I expected the emotional impact of losing my brother would hit me soon enough, together with the questions regarding how long he had lived and whether he had suffered. Yet in some ways the certainty that it would have happened removed any apprehension about hearing confirmation. Before, it had been just him and me. Then there had been progressively less of him. Now it was just me... alone.

After checking into my expansive hotel room, I continued to read the orientation manual we had been given. It informed me that my concerns about the underground tunnel I had just travelled through were unfounded. Being situated on a geological fault line mattered no more. At the centre of the city, buried deep within the earth, was a stabilising brace, protecting its citizens. Looking out of the open hotel room window at the crystal blue bay, I was struck by the freshness of the air I was breathing. The water glittered in the sunlight and in the distance, I could hear voices, but unusually, no sounds of traffic. I had never been to San Francisco before. The landscape I saw before me was notable, not for its modernity but for the serenity it presented. The relative silence was not what I would have expected of a major city. Rather than being eerie, I found it strangely calming.

I drank some water from the minibar. It tasted delicious and crisp. Reading more about the historical, technological and political changes of the last twenty years whetted my appetite for venturing into the hub of the city. However as I checked the GPS on my tablet and saw the distance from my hotel to the Golden Gate Bridge, a wave of exhaustion swept over me and I realised that it was time to get some rest. I entered the shower and after being doused from all sides with a fine mist of hot water followed by a cold spray, I allowed myself to be blow-dried before retiring to collapse on the king-size bed. Automatically the lights begin to dim and the windows darkened as I entered a tranquil sleep.

It was noon the following day when I finally arose. My slumber was broken gently, with a steady pulse of light emerging from the clock on my bedside table. I opened my eyes with a fresh head and rapidly clearing conscience. Padding across to the cupboard, I examined the clothes that had been placed inside for me. The shirt and trousers appeared to have been made of the same material as the underwear: lightweight, micro-fibre fabric that felt like silk.

I was standing observing myself in the mirror with a newfound sense of optimism when the television screen lit up and an electronic voice announced that I had a visitor in reception.

'Who is it?' I asked warily.

'Your brother, Mr Demille: Ryan.'

Stunned, I didn't speak for several moments until the television patiently reminded me that my guest was waiting.

'Send him up, please.'

It was only two to three minutes until the knock on my door but it felt like an age. During this time, I had sat on the edge of my bed, knuckles gripping the edges.

How was it possible that he had lived this long?

After the knock was repeated, I rose to open the door, my hands trembling. Instinctively I looked down only to see a narrow waist, slim denim clad legs and brown loafers. Confused I cast my eyes up to stare into a smiling face I barely recognised: one I vaguely recalled in its younger form before the degenerative effects of motor neurone disease had contorted it, wiping away all trace of hope and confidence, both qualities which were now restored in the radiant and healthy adult I saw before me.

'I can't believe it's you,' marvelled Ryan.

I grabbed him in a tight embrace which he returned, patting my back comfortingly.

After the tears had been wiped away and I had recaptured enough presence of mind to welcome him into the room, I poured us each a glass of champagne and we sat, laughing and joking. At first I skirted around the obvious question, afraid that I would break the illusion, until finally I could wait no longer.

'How long have you been like this?'

Ryan's face became serious as he answered. 'I was still in a pretty bad way for a long time after you disappeared. The carer I had at the time hung around for a bit after the money ran out, but eventually the house got sold and I was placed in a home. I was scared. If it had been possible, I think I would have ended it.

'Then about thirteen years ago, some people came to collect me and brought me to San Francisco. There was a biotechnology company specialising in degenerative diseases and they wanted me to take part in trials for the stem cell therapy treatment they were developing. There were some false starts but over the course of the next two years I began to find it a little easier to talk, to move my neck and then, well...' he held out his arms and looked at me meaningfully. 'I owe them everything. After I was fully recovered I picked up my studies from where I left off and now I'm working for them in their operations division.'

'How on earth did a company in San Francisco come across you in a London care home?'

'I think it best he tell you directly.'

'Who?'

'Jared Rathbone.'

I knew that this had all been too easy.

***

The journey up to Laurel Heights was above ground at my insistence. I needed the fresh air and didn't want to lose sight of the sky. The cab we took was a driverless Tesla which moved with a gentle purr, the navigation system pointing out places of interest as we progressed. Ryan spoke little as we travelled, allowing me to gaze out of the window.

The revelation of whom we were about to meet made me wonder again whether I was dreaming: Jared Rathbone, the billionaire founder of PureGen, a company that had started out as a clean energy venture before expanding into environmental solutions and biotechnology. A man cited as being pivotal in reducing the world's reliance on fossil fuels, making clean drinking water available to all reaches of the developing world, extending the average human lifespan by fifteen years and narrowing the difference in human mortality levels between the developed and developing world.

The man I'd been sent to kill.

I didn't believe in coincidences. Not only had a person I'd been despatched to assassinate twenty years ago managed to turn the world around during my extended hiatus, but during that time he had also happened across my brother and cured him of a crippling disease. The more I thought about it the more likely it seemed that any minute, I was going to blink and find myself back in the cabin of Flight 008 preparing to land in San Francisco. This surreal drama was probably just my conscience trying to ease me out of the course of action I'd committed to.

I looked across at Ryan watching me. It had been so good to see him this way. I stared intently, wanting to sear the image in my mind. My questions to him were partially driven by the desire to hear his voice, clear and uninterrupted by the rasping croak by which it had previously been encumbered.

'What's he like?'

'Jared? You'd think he'd be this hyperactive guy who gets up at 5am each day and is constantly on his mobile. He's intelligent without a doubt. But he comes across as something of a daydreamer. I think you'll like him.'

The cab began to slow down, eventually stopping outside a mansion block at the top of a pristine road. Ryan pressed his thumb briefly against the panel on the dashboard and as it flashed to record payment, the doors opened to allow us out. After Ryan had his iris scanned by a small box to the right of the front door, we entered a marble hallway with a lift at the far end, which we took up to the top floor. We alighted on to a vast, sparsely furnished space. At one side was a well-stacked bar with a couple of stools whilst at the other end, a chaise-longue faced a screen that covered the majority of the wall, relaying multiple feeds from Bloomberg, CNN and the BBC. Surrounding us was a wraparound floor-to-ceiling window, offering spectacular views of San Francisco. Standing in front of the panel and looking out at the Golden Gate Bridge with his profile to us was Jared Rathbone.

He turned as we approached, greeting us with a welcoming smile. He looked young, barely changed from the photos of him I had seen in Tokyo. He reached out a hand to me.

'Howard, welcome. It's good to finally meet you. I imagine the last twenty-four hours must have felt quite surreal. How are you feeling? Has it sunk in yet?'

'I've slept through most of the day,' I confessed, disarmed by his easy manner. 'But it's all starting to become more familiar.'

'Good to hear,' he saw my eyes darting behind him to the view. It's something else, isn't it? On my busiest days, it soothes me to spend time looking out across the bay. Why don't you spend a few moments taking it in while I fix you a drink? Ryan, do you want to give me a hand?'

He headed across to the bar with Ryan in tow. Deciding that there was little I could do other than see where this sequence of events would lead, I followed his suggestion and paced the floor, appreciating the city skyline and wondering how my own modest London suburb looked, twenty years on.

'What happened to our old home?' I called back to Ryan.

'Still exactly as it was,' replied Ryan, grinning. 'Since I started working, I was able to buy a place here without needing to sell up. I still go back every now and again. I guess you could say it's a shrine to the way things were. Listen, I've got a couple of calls to make. They won't take long, but I'm going to pop out for a few minutes while you guys get acquainted. When we get back, we should go for an early dinner.'

'Sounds like a plan,' concurred Jared, before I could say anything. He walked over to hand me a Long Island Iced Tea, watching me as I hesitantly waved goodbye to Ryan.

'Your brother has been an invaluable member of my company these last couple of years. I've never seen someone with his level of energy before.'

'Thank you for everything you've done for him. I still can't believe it's the same person I'm looking at.'

I felt like a fraud saying this. I was intensely grateful, but could barely look him in the eye, without the images flashing in my mind of that room back in Tokyo, surrounded by unsmiling faces repeating instructions at me: how I would find him; where to attack; how to escape...

'You're very welcome. Ryan's progress even took me by surprise. I'll never forget how it felt to see him walk unaided.'

'How exactly did you find him? There must have been plenty of candidates here in the US. How did he land on your radar?'

Jared nodded. 'I guess you could call it a side-effect of your flight's disappearance. As you can imagine, it got a lot of news coverage. I learned that one of the missing passengers was a journalist who had a meeting scheduled with me for an article about my clean energy venture.'

I nodded, remembering the ruse that had been concocted for the meeting.

'Around the same time, I got a call from one of my team regarding a beta test on a side project we were running in the field of electronic surveillance. He'd been working on a piece of software that would combine data from various sources: CCTV, email, mobile telecommunications, whilst maintaining an encryption that would only unlock itself and reveal the source if it detected any patterns that increased the probability of specific stress scenarios. We'd been working with sponsorship from the NSA on it and several interesting patterns came up. We shared the results of one discovery with them: it caused the opening of an investigation which triggered a major upheaval in our government. Another lead indicated that my name had been flagged in communications between employees of a private security company and several major oil and pharmaceutical firms... and that it also came up in a video recording that one of those employees sent from their mobile phone to a local area network the day before Flight JNS 008 set off from Tokyo.'

At this point, Jared tapped his smartwatch and gestured to the television behind us.

'I just want you to know before you watch this that I haven't shown it to any law enforcement authorities. Only a handful of trusted employees of mine have seen it.'

The screen flickered before displaying a scene in a dimly lit room. Several men were seated across a table littered with photographs and sheets of paper. The picture was shaky as if the recording was being made surreptitiously. I blinked, a sheen of sweat forming on my brow as I stared at the sequence, barely hearing the words being spoken. I was staring at myself on the screen, at the head of the table, looking uncomfortably at photographs of Jared, shortly before my flight to San Francisco.

As I trembled, I felt Jared's hand on my shoulder. I looked up at him to see a face devoid of anger.

'Mr Rathbone,' I blurted. 'Please allow me to explain.'

'It's okay.'

'I'm sorry?'

Jared smiled sympathetically.

'I'm saying I understand what happened. They looked for someone who was desperate, short on money, with little family and an urgent need – to support a brother wholly dependent upon him. They made an offer that he couldn't refuse and made sure he realised that to refuse would likely endanger them both. The fact one of them recorded it indicated they were planning on using it against you further down the line. They did all this merely to get rid of me because they thought I threatened their livelihood. Why it didn't occur to them to invest in my venture and do something constructive to help this planet rather than just focus on profit, I'll never know. In any case, they were too late. Shortly after the success of the work I did with the NSA, the government got more interested in the other ventures I was running, provided me with the funding I needed and things moved much more quickly. We got a breakthrough in developing a scalable clean energy solution for the planet and with all the publicity we were receiving, I became far too high profile for anyone to risk trying anything against me.

'After we'd beefed personnel up at the company and I had the opportunity to expand into some of the other areas I was interested in, I wanted to find out what had happened to Ryan and help him if possible. After all, if it hadn't been for you being roped into trying to kill me, you'd never have been on that plane and he would still have had a brother to look after him. The rest is... well, it's history for me but news to you.'

I stared at him in disbelief. 'You mean to say that you don't think I should be punished for what I was going to do?'

'Frankly Howard, I doubt very much that you would have followed through with murder. I ran facial and voice analysis on that video and spoke to people who knew you, including Ryan of course. The profile I built up indicates someone who was more likely to report the matter to the authorities once he had the chance to think the matter over. I suspect it's why you missed your initial flight out of Tokyo and had to be placed on 008 – to buy yourself some time. No, in my opinion, and based upon the simulation I ran on this scenario, you just never got the chance to steer yourself back on the right track and I will never hold that against you. The only thing I ask of you is that you make the most of this opportunity to start afresh and make a life for yourself in the same way that your brother has done. That and one other favour...'

'Of course – anything.'

'It so happens that I own the San Francisco Chronicle,' said Jared, beaming. 'And the editor would be overjoyed if you'd be so kind as to grant him an exclusive first interview.'

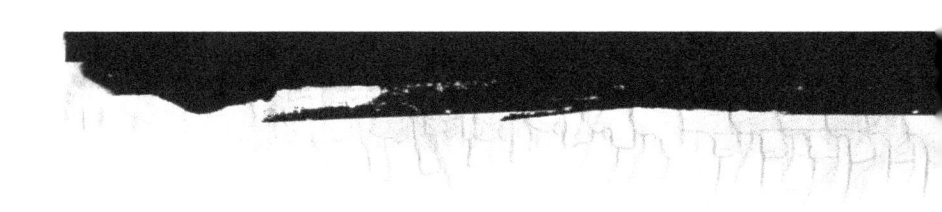

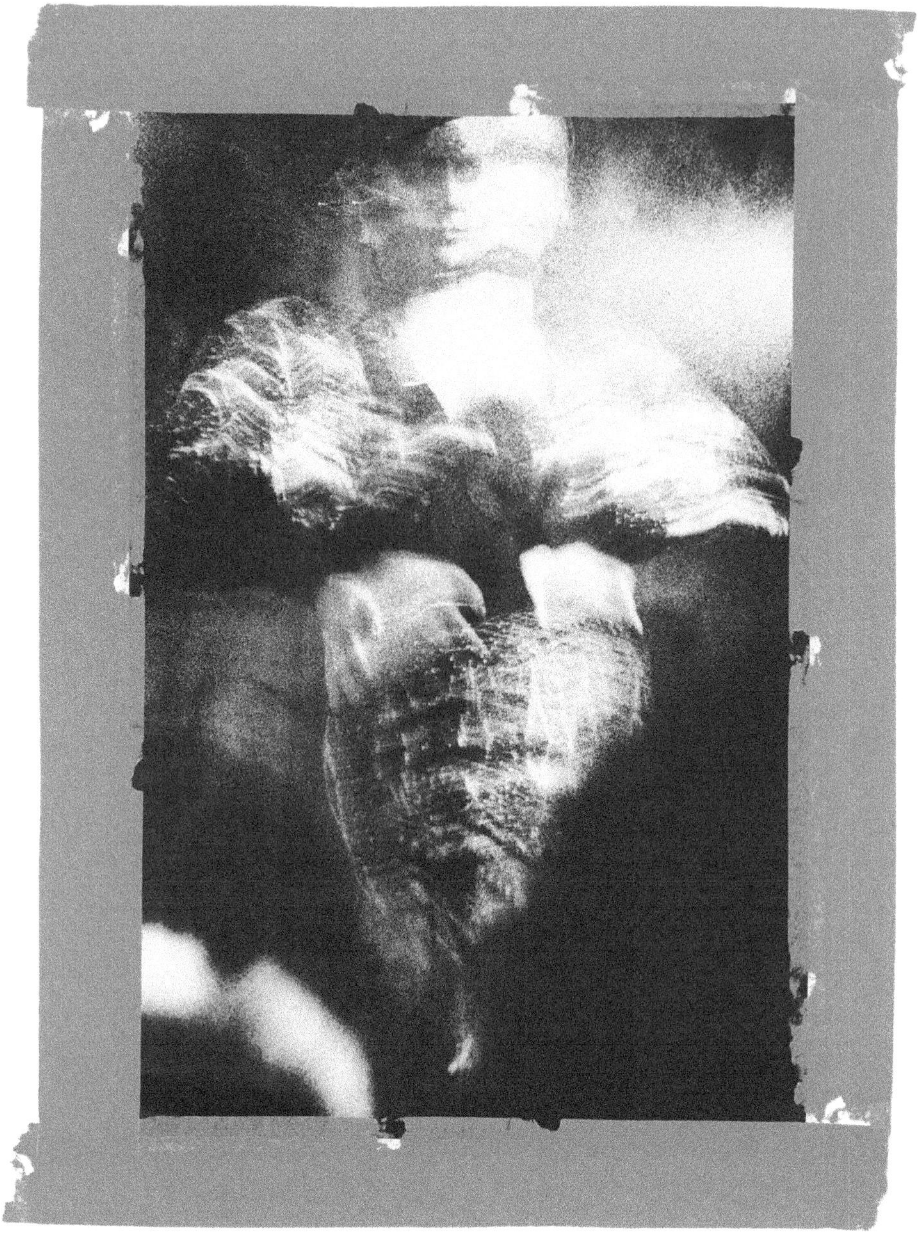

ALL I SEE

by Anna Pen

Trump is on TV in the living room. I hear him saying, 'All options are on the table.'
We are having breakfast in the kitchen, looking out at the birds pecking at our birdfeeder.
'Bird eat yummy eat,' Marie says as she licks and sucks all the butter from her toast.
Trump continues, 'They best not make any more threats to the US. They will be met with fire and fury like the world has never seen.'
My period has stopped. It didn't really start. A couple of brown spots but nothing else and then four and a half days with nothing. This is exactly how Marie began.
She holds her arms out to get down and I lift her from her booster seat. She starts busying, taking things out of the kitchen drawers.
'A book and a shick a bye,' she tells me and then wanders through the patio door into the garden and begins clipping the hedges with a tin opener.
Our beautiful world, coming to an end.

***

When she is down for her nap, I listen to music that makes me ache inside with burning nostalgia for all that was: the hit of dry smoke as we walked into a club, feeling that rush, all of us together dancing with every part of ourselves, dew on the grass as we walked back in the early morning from a night out – all of the beautiful connections between music and minds and sounds.

Second child, second coming, second chance. Seconds left. Words play through my mind as I feel that desperate dread inside, like a groaning, anxious homesickness.

I scroll down the newsfeed on my phone and it tells me that we cannot expect Trump to act with responsibility.

After her nap, I go through the usual coat struggle with Marie and we finally get out to the park. The turning leaves smell so heavy and beautiful that it hits my heart and tears spring to my eyes. Mark will be back soon. My womb is closing around a secret like a fist.

***

But afternoon turns to night and his keys haven't clicked in the keyhole.

When Marie is in bed I call his phone eight times, then I pour myself a glass of wine and gulp half of it down before chucking it into the sink. I make mint tea and start calling round friends and family to see if anyone has heard from Mark. The only person that seems to take his disappearance half seriously is his sister Jean.

'I can't get hold of him either.'

'The thing is, I know whatever he's doing he would let me know because of Marie, with everything going on.'

'Going on? Is everything okay? But yep... it is strange. I'll let you know straight away if I hear from him, okay?'

I put down the phone and look out at the lines of drizzle hitting the streetlamp's orange glow.

A trickle of dread hits me near my backbone, where our tails used to be. I become aware of what has happened. I feel his absence and the turn in our reality hits me. He hasn't turned his phone off, he has turned his life off. Bastard.

***

I stay in the kitchen all night, and then it is daytime and Marie is up again, with her fresh little missions. Still the TV news is rolling in from the living room, words and words and words talking about the 'tense situation'. No one discusses the specifics about who will die first, how many in the initial blasts, how many more from ruptured insides, murder, and suicide. It is obvious everyone will just talk about the threat until one of them has pressed the button and it has all happened and we will be so flooded with disbelief and shock and death and panic that we will have no way to discuss our options rationally.

I have done the right thing to insist on this house on Factory Lane, with the air raid shelter at the end of the garden, even though it is more than we can really afford. Maybe he has ended his life because he can't handle me being right. Despite these years of loving me, he always hated how I can see it all coming. He just plunged us all into violent outbursts of silence for days on end, his secret fear coiled around us like a python.

There will have been a moment for him at the sanctuary yesterday when he will have stopped still – halfway through teaching primary kids about badgers and blue tits or mid-sandwich in the staff hut. At that moment the truth would have suddenly poured into him like wet concrete.

He would have planned his ending there and then. He would have convinced himself that he was going into a long hibernation. They will find him somewhere, curled up in a ball like a hedgehog, my man with the soft curls. When I first saw him we edged closer, danced together by the speakers, being pulled into a deep, frenzied vortex of happiness. After the club, we sat on my friend's living room floor, talking until morning, steadily filling each other up with hope. Mark, with whom my life rolled on, propelled forwards by his quiet voice and loud green eyes.

My entire being yearns for those perfect days that are lost forever: our picnics in parks, afternoons drinking beers at Keith's wine bar, more nights out filled with ecstasy and music and love followed by those perfect days after, where we just stayed in bed and let that love evaporate into the air with the sweat from our bodies. Somehow in those days we just knew more beauty was around the corner, but we never really stopped to notice it, as if we knew that if we stared it in the face it would turn away from us.

I stand in the kitchen, holding the edge of the kitchen table, remembering that February walk along the beach, his proposal against the steel grey sky with freezing spray hitting our faces, a simple ceremony in the woods, summers of camping and BBQs and swims in the river. Six months in South East Asia, crystal sharp moments of stunned disbelief at our luck. Then Marie.

I know he loved her like I do. I watched him revelling in her simple pleasures. I saw his face light up when she 'mmm'd' and 'ahhh'd' over the soft surfaces of a peeled boiled egg. He brought her upstairs every evening to let her spend as much time as she wanted throwing things in a running bath. How could he let it go so easily? He has quit his life in a panic, like a frantic push of the button to stop the fire alarm when the toast is burning. If only he had been with me in understanding and accepting what's coming and had helped me prepare for it. Instead he became disgusted by me and my acceptance of it.

'You are ruining our lives with your weird shit and it's not fair on anyone. You need to get it sorted. It's fucking selfish.'

That's the last thing he said to me before he left yesterday morning. At the time, it didn't bother me. He has been saying that to me pretty much every day for the last few months, whilst I have been preparing.

We have our bunker. Out of everyone in the world, we have the highest chance of survival. This obviously did not comfort him enough.

Five months ago, millions were made homeless in New Orleans as the first of the five major hurricanes hit. Two months later it was Beijing under water and by the end of last year huge hurricanes had hit Cuba and the Philippines. Indescribable amounts of houses and cars and trees litter the world – dead bodies under water, millions of people sick, their loved ones lost. In the middle of it all, Trump rose, puffed out his chest, turned the corner of his mouth down and began belching out his yellow warnings to North Korea.

I told Mark to admit that this was the beginning of the end. I tried to make him see that it was time to stop forgetting it all, time to bring our heads up from our everyday lives and focus on planning our survival. I felt the animal instinct to protect and I was sick of him badgering on with things as if there was nothing to worry about.

I knew he did worry. I watched him sitting and staring at a wall, willing himself to put socks on and go to work. Despite being so frustrated with him, I mostly just wanted to envelop him and take his fear away. All I could do was press myself physically to him, to take his mind off things in a clumsy effort to break through to him. I assume that one episode of this physical envelopment has led to the tightening in my womb and the heat in my breasts.

I knew he had not been sleeping well, for a long while. What about me, though? I have had a million sleepless nights. My eyeballs have dried out so much and I have become so prickly from the exhaustion that I have stopped eye contact, phone calls to friends, listening to music and reading for pleasure. The constant threats facing my baby since she entered the world have turned me inside out – I could never walk up the steps in town or over a bridge with her without visualizing her falling, head to concrete or body sinking swiftly into water, far too quickly for me to catch her. If not an accident, then the fear that she will be stunted or not hit her milestones. I became fixated with reading all the forum threads of the disasters that come up in real life to some poor other mother somewhere: 'my son has turned blue, had a febrile convulsion, choked on a grape, fell down the stairs, has a fever that won't go down.' I felt like it must surely be her time, that she would not possibly survive this treacherous infancy. It was an impossible notion that something would not go wrong and we would not lose her – of course she would break or slip away and it would be all our fault. She would be gone. We would not be able to carry on.

She didn't die though, she is standing millimetres away from the TV screen watching Bing and eating occasional handfuls of buttered egg from the breakfast plate I have put on the coffee table in the living room.

Despite what is coming, we have more of a chance than most people. We have our concrete tunnel of protection. He gave up too easily but we are still here.

We go out to Thingamabobs for a camping light and stove and then the supermarket for a pregnancy test and tinned foods.

Marie stands on her step at the sink playing with the toothbrushes as I do the test. The stick doesn't reveal anything that I did not already feel deep inside me, but now at least we can go down into that bunker with sure knowledge of what our personal circumstances are. One gone, one to come. If we have tins and warmth and light and safety I will have proved him wrong. We will survive.

I make Marie spaghetti with almost half a block of cheese on top and we eat it straight from the pan. It seems ridiculous that the bomb will drop, that people's faces will fall off, that we will all be sick and die.

I leave the pan in the sink and Marie follows me into the February drizzle, dragging her play pushchair with her battered Bing toy in. I heave our last few boxes into the bunker and then we close the door behind us. I turn on our battery-powered light and radio and listen for more from Trump.

'The fury is coming and they should all take cover. No one should underestimate the force that I can promise is coming to them. Nobody not ever, never forget the force.'

I shut the door. We cuddle up on the big armchair I have bought especially for this place and read stories. After that we get out playdough and we while the time away until it is time for Marie to sleep. It is important for us to stick to our timings and routines. Her body is soon a warm deadweight in my arms and she is that familiar sleeping being of mine, the elfin spirit of a human that I have created.

I breathe in and out and imagine us all unfolding like flowers, me and my buds. When we come out of here, who knows what will have happened with the world, but we will be in it and I will add to it and we will respect it and be gentle with what's left.

Muffled shouts come closer. It's him calling us. He's trying to claw his way back into our world but it's too late. He has made his decision.

The shout gets closer. He is calling our names. At first, I think she won't wake up, but then she does and she pulls out of my arms. When I put her down she runs to the end of the tunnel shelter, towards the muffled sound of him calling our names. I turn the radio up so that we can't hear him.

'Daddy?'

'No, it's okay Marie, come here, sit with me.'

On the radio is a gardening programme, I turn it up loud and distract Marie with her milk and hold her to my shoulder, bouncing her up and down like I did when she was tiny.

'It's important to get the buds in early and then leave them to it, you can cover them if needs be but even if left, they are sturdy and you should see shoots after about three months.'

After a while the shouts stop. He must have gone back to where he knows he has taken himself. Away from this world, away from us.

Marie is asleep again on my shoulder and I turn the radio off, drinking in the silence, just her breathing and the underground pulses of our hearts beating together.

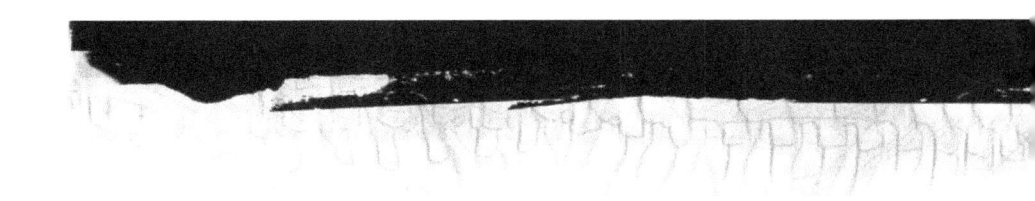

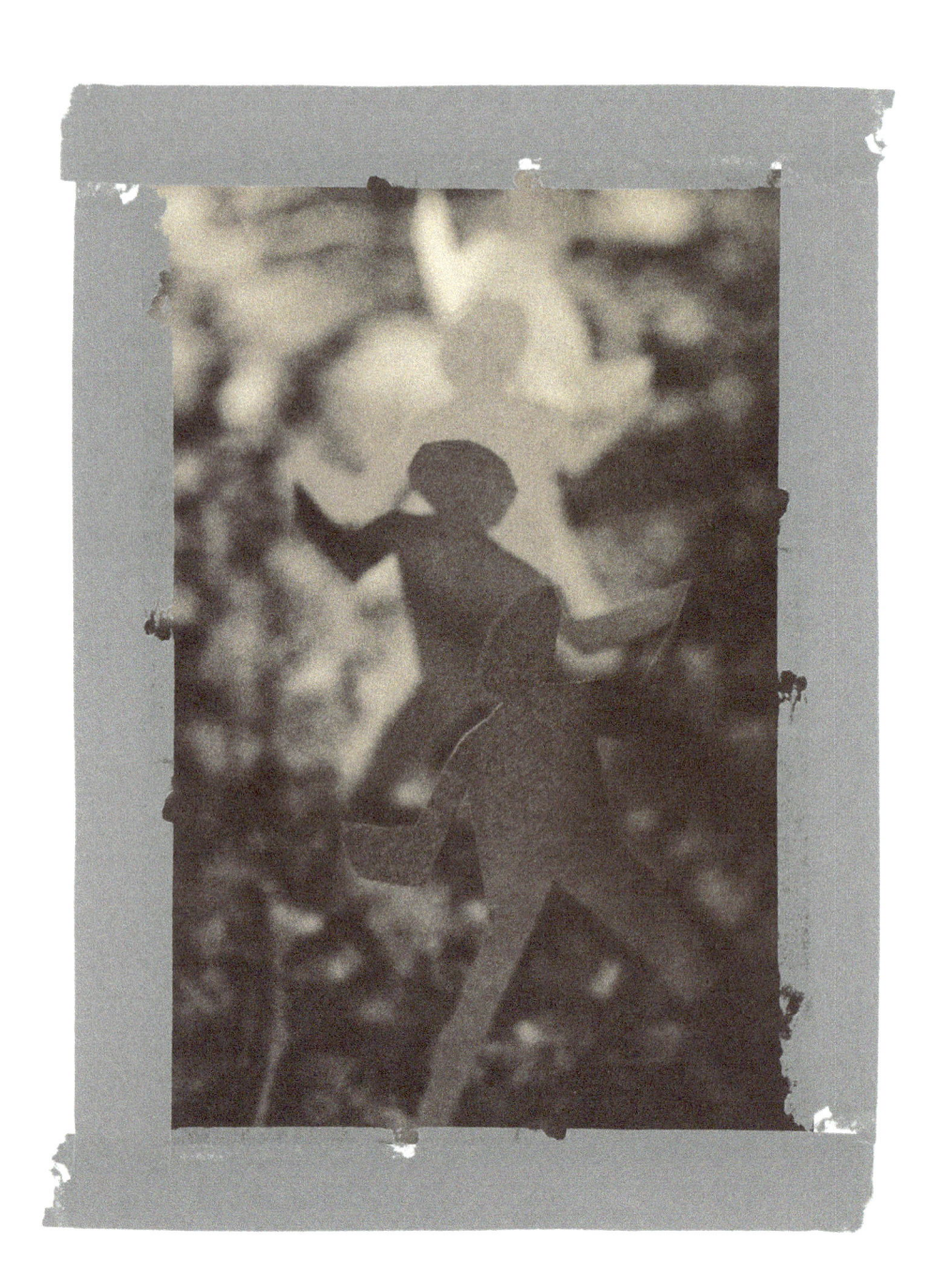

THE TURKEY IN THE BOOT

by Emily White

Now it's such a quiet house. And I do dust the piano. Dad pays for it to be tuned once a year – sends his man over. I sit on the sofa to the sound of his tuning. 'Bing, bing bip! Bing, bing bip! Bing, bing' – I feel such a profound stillness in the sound. Like listening to a drip shape a rock.

My ears ring – a hiss that arrived the year you left. Or maybe, because I am no longer listening for you, I hear it.

I try to imagine this room as it was that year. That incredible final Christmas, when you inspired us to so many parties. When the cocktails swam into the room in a haze of basil and crushed ice.

Liberated from hope. Our hearts soared with the freedom.

Gradually I am throwing out the exotic bottles from that frenzy. Some terrible cherry thing got sent down the sink – but the tequila went to a good home.

The dog's limbs are twitching as she dreams. The house sighs too.

It began with the turkey in the boot.

Even before – it started with our realisation; this was the Christmas we got to choose.

First the decorations – exquisite paper chains made by women in India, sent in brown boxes from the Amnesty warehouse. They were draped across the dusty ceiling – bypassing damp patches and flaking paint. Then the tree was dug up from the garden. Hilariously big. You were site manager for the front room. 'We need to leave room for Pam to play the piano' you said from your elegant top-range wheelchair, one hand clutching the cocktail. Once the giant tree was wedged in the corner we collaborated on tinsel, me threshing amongst the branches as you masterminded the artistry – the glass, paper, and pottery from the accumulated years. You drew the line at the bread and boiled-sweet church windows that were a grim dusty heap amongst the treasures. These examples of nephew art were relegated to the compost.

Three parties were planned – thirty people crammed into the cottage, awash with gifts of fantastic wine, cheap cider and local beer. Karl with his piercings, Jon from the Parkinson's club, Glen the elegant dancer, who had us whirling around the room, and the shy children from next door – witnesses to the secret side of the human story. The flight times from New York, Aberdeen, Inverness were all part of our schedules. Extra bedding planned, duvet covers laundered ready. Guests came in droves to pack the house in all its corners – dog circling in endless welcome.

***

Christmas Eve and the dented Ford opened its doors to take us to London for Midnight Mass. In it we folded the wheelchair, the lung suction machine – the surgical gloves, the sterile packs – spare tracheotomy tubes. Why was all that so funny? But it was – as we stuffed medication, spare clothes just in case, a pile of instruments, three guests in the back, and you – cheeks bunched in a smile, in the front. I relished the drag of the absurdly loaded vehicle. Just before we left, the turkey was delivered. Didn't fit in the fridge! 'Boot of my car' says you – so it was well wrapped to avoid the casual oil cans – and the great beast was laid to rest in the grandeur of a blue Jag.

And so the triumphal party glided through the centre of London, thronged with Christmas Eve shoppers. 'Look! Buckingham Palace! Helloo Queenie!' shouted the Scottish nationalists with delight from the back of the car. 'Oh my' was the Brooklyn professor's sigh as The

Natural History Museum, St James's Park, and Harrods sailed past the windows. You put your thumb over the speaking tube so we could share the sound of the wheezing and the bubbles.

You feasted on Turkish prawns and mouth-watering bites. The restaurant opened a side door to accommodate the unexpected wheelchair – how each exquisite mouthful was relished and chosen with care. How the taste plates kept coming, and miraculously you ate them, to the pride and delight of us all. Hours later, shiny faced, fuzzy with the last meal of a lifetime you made your royal progress into the dark expanse of Westminster Cathedral for Midnight Mass.

In the hours of music and prayers to come there was plenty of swearing from the Scots and bladder concerns from anyone who had had a beer. But there was a thread of something else from high in the choir down to the congregation where you sat listening for my music in the darkness. For two hours I sent my messages to you in that great hall – an expanse of church black. Hushed, full of people, and all those listeners on the BBC.

Then there was the ridiculous journey home through the darkest hours of Christmas morning. You all filled the car with stories to keep me awake, already solidifying the narrative for the years ahead. The amazing waiters, the delicious food, the drunk mother and daughter next to you in the Cathedral – the Latin genius behind, poking everyone in the back to stand and sit in the service – the explosion of 'Fer Fooks sake!' from Mr Scotland on the ninetieth Latin prayer – only for him to remember in a rush he was live on national radio. And how you were wheeled up for a blessing and got two hands and reverence and care. And Pam a mere cursory 'Yep blessing on you too madam' – the sexist bastards.

And the singing began. Carols – belted at the top of the five voices as we trundled through the blackened country lanes. Pam kicked the driver's seat in time to the music – windows all down – gales thrashing in our faces. 'Glo—ooo—ooooooo-oooo-ree-ya!' we yelled as we descended into the town at 4.38am.

And the next day was your Christmas day. You masterminded our feast – with a team of us sous chefs. This was the Christmas I saw for the first time my mum cry with laughter. Call My Bluff. I know you won – best liar of the lot. That was the Christmas I got a group selfie of us all – red-cheeked with champagne – and we had coffee in the garden in the snow, holding hot water bottles.

    Pam did play the piano – Keith banged a bottle as percussion, and we all sang.

***

Here in my tinnitus hiss I sit in the stillness and people this little world again, with you. And fill my ears with your singing.

'Bing Bing Bip! Bing Bing Bip! Bing Bing'

Christmas. This year I expect I will be in the office room at Mum and Dad's again, on a mattress. And all the family together.

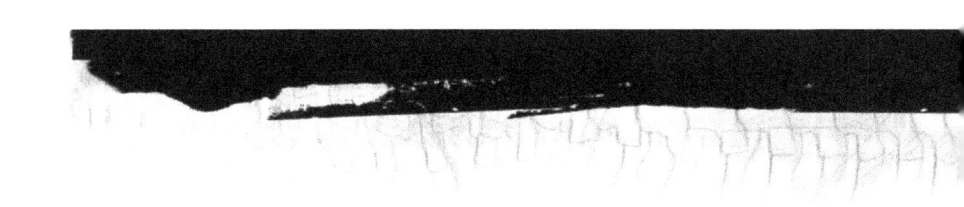

ABOUT THE CONTRIBUTORS

Nicola Cassidy is a writer and blogger from Co. Louth, Ireland. She published her debut historical fiction novel *December Girl* with Bombshell Books in late 2017 and it became an Amazon bestseller in 2018. She has signed a three book deal with Irish Publisher Poolbeg Books and will release her second historical fiction novel in summer 2019. When she's not writing and researching novels, Nicola blogs at www.ladynicci.com, an award-nominated lifestyle blog, and tends to her young family.

Michael Coolwood is a male author who writes feminist Science Fiction and Fantasy novels. Most, such as the recently released steampunk murder mystery *Drown the Witch* and the comedy of errors *Confessions of a Gentleman Arachnid,* are informed by his experiences of living with depression, anxiety and fatigue.

Pam Corsie's U3A Creative Writing Group meets once a week for mutual encouragement in following their writing dream. They have self-published an anthology of short stories, *Ladies in Beach Huts* and are working on their second, *It All Happens in Dorset*, for publication this Christmas. Pam also has a first in Writing Magazine, a shortlisted story soon to be published in an anthology by Eyelands publishers, several 'honourable mentions' in various competitions, 3rd prize in a limerick competition and an article in *Cycling* Magazine. She self-published a family history beginning in the mid 1800s, *From Little Acorns*, narrated by a daughter from each generation.

Claire Goodman is a writer, living and working in South East London. This is her first published short story. Her work focusses on the nuances of everyday life and is often based around giving voice to emotional territories, that concern more vulnerable members of society.

Jamie Harding is a quality control officer who lives in Hertfordshire with his wife Jo and their dog Dave. His experience of living with depression and chronic pain informs his writing, as does witnessing the lives of people close to him with serious psychiatric illnesses, having seen the stigmatism and downright assault on one's mind and sense of self that these conditions can bring about. He reads a lot, and writes a lot more, having dabbled in freelance copy-writing and penned jokes for BBC Radio. He regularly writes for the online news satire site *NewsThump* and is currently putting the finishing touches on his debut novel, *the Shadow Author*.

Jim Knight is a writer from the West Midlands. His fiction has been published elsewhere and is usually of the dirty realist and stream of consciousness variety - he is currently working on a project of novel length. His story 'For Steve', details a few of his great-uncles' last days; as well as some reflections on American society from an English socialist's perspective, he thinks his uncle would appreciate this. Jim would like to highlight the detrimental effect of austerity on disabled people and the huge rise in suicides - it is no coincidence and it can be stopped.

Sarah Longthorne is a prose, games, and screenplay writer living in Cambridge. She graduated from the University of East Anglia in 2014 with a first-class degree in Scriptwriting and Performance following a ten-year battle with depression and bulimia, which informs many of her stories. You can find more information about Sarah and her work at **www.sarahlongthorne.com**.

Alison McCrossan lives in Ireland. She has been published in Crannog Magazine and Foxglove Journal.

Roland Miles used to be an English and Drama teacher, working extensively with children in devised theatre. He now sells second-hand books. He has an MA in Creative Writing from the University of Sussex. He has just completed a collection of short stories about life in schools, as yet unpublished, and a book entitled *Chaucer the Actor: The Canterbury Tales as Performance Art.*

Diane L. Miller grew up in western Pennsylvania, USA and studied in Canada on a Fulbright Scholarship. After suffering with celiac disease for decades, she was finally diagnosed five years ago. For the past nineteen years, she has worked as a writer/editor in the technology and consulting industries. Prior to that, she worked as a journalist and has written for several business and technology publications including Wired. She lives in London with her husband and two daughters and writes fiction on the sly.

Shirley Muir is a medieval re-enactor, molecular biologist, tarot reader and writer of fiction and poetry. She spends her time between the east coast of Scotland and the Turkish mountains, where she watches the International Space Station streak across the backdrop of the Milky Way. She won the inaugural Crediton Festival short story competition in 2015 and has been published in the UK, Australia and the USA. Her work has appeared in The Eildon Tree, Whortleberry Press, InfectiveInk, Caesura, Bunbury, and the Henshaw anthology.

A note from Bea Mulder:
Hello   :)
I am a thirteen-year-old artist and writer living in a woodland with my mother, brother, three strange cats and a mad spaniel. For a homework project in Year 8 English, we were asked to write 500 words-within the theme 'Feeling the Pressure'. Instead I found myself working on it for six weeks and by the end it was more than 5000 words long! I'd never written anything with a deeper, more mature meaning, but once I started I couldn't stop. I think that I was subconsciously very influenced by having just lost my granny, Susan, who was bipolar. A

general awareness of mental health inspired me, but the story is not autobiographical.
Have a nice day,
B

Neel Patel was born in London in 1979. He was educated at the City of London School and graduated from the London School of Economics before qualifying as a chartered accountant. His subsequent career in finance has included spells abroad in Budapest and Dublin. An avid reader of fiction, autobiography and history, he has written creatively since childhood and has a particular interest in stories that explore the achievements of the human spirit in the face of adversity. He currently lives and works in London.

Anna Pen has recently returned from an eight year adventure in Cambodia, and is now back in the UK and training as a secondary school English teacher in Essex. She has spent a number of years working within in the special educational needs and disabilities department in secondary schools, working with fantastic young people who remain true to themselves and determined despite facing massive emotional and physical challenges every day.

Emily White was married to the poet Brian Nisbet. She had great pleasure in learning about writing from him. After his death from MSA in 2015, she has enjoyed writing - knowing he would be relishing the attempts. She won this year's Brian Nisbet Poetry award based in his home town of Huntly. Being alongside Brian as his illness took hold, until his eventual death at home, was a life changing honour that taught her much about grace and generosity of heart.

Dr Tansy Spinks is an artist, sound artist and educator currently involved in creating sound works for spaces using improvisation with conventional and non-conventional sound making devices. She has a PhD in Sound Art, an MA in Photography from the Royal College of Art, a BA in Fine Art from Leeds Polytechnic and is a Licentiate of the Guildhall

School of Music (violin). Her photographic work is in The Museum of Fine Art, Houston and the National Media Museum, Bradford, now at the V&A. She has exhibited nationally and internationally. She has taught and been an external examiner at many art schools nationally and is currently Senior Lecturer in Fine Art, running the MA Fine Art at Middlesex University. She lives and works in South London.
Contact details:
http://www.tansyspinks.com
contact@tansyspinks.com or t.spinks@mdx.ac.uk

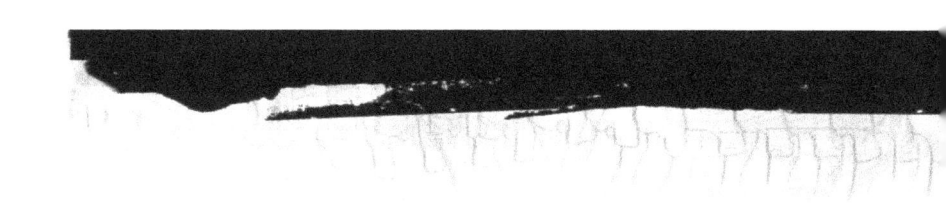

ABOUT THE JUDGES

James Scott is a semi-retired surgeon and is currently the Emeritus Editor of an Orthopaedic Surgical Journal. He was the founding Chairman of the Arts Project at the Chelsea and Westminster Hospital when it opened in 1993. He is the author of a recent book about the sculpture of Kenneth Armitage.

Katie Isbester Ph.D. is is the founder and Editor-in-Chief of Claret Press, an artisan publishing house. As an author she has published with academic presses and commercial magazines, including The Times Literary Supplement. As a publisher, she has produced a dozen fiction and non-fiction books. The achievements of Claret Press's books include being award-winnning finalists, being translated into German, and being endorsed by international best-selling authors.

Sarah Gray is notorious for her supernatural, psychological thrillers. Each of her characters is forced to endure their own personal haunting: domestic abuse, anxiety and depression, repressed sexuality – there's an apparition for every condition. In a past life Sarah was a television editor and studied literature and most styles of writing. She is also the creator of her own short films. Master of the short story, her two collections *Surface Tension* and *Half Life* are replete with curious stories that cause disquiet, heartache and a thrilling sting of pleasure. Coming in summer 2019, *Urban Creatures* is set to complete her uniquely dark trilogy. Sarah was diagnosed with Motor Neurone Disease in October 2015 and since then has been skilfully learning how to adapt to

disability and grappling with a reduced lifespan. This has tinged her work a shade darker. For more information about Sarah and her books, visit
www.racontesse.com.

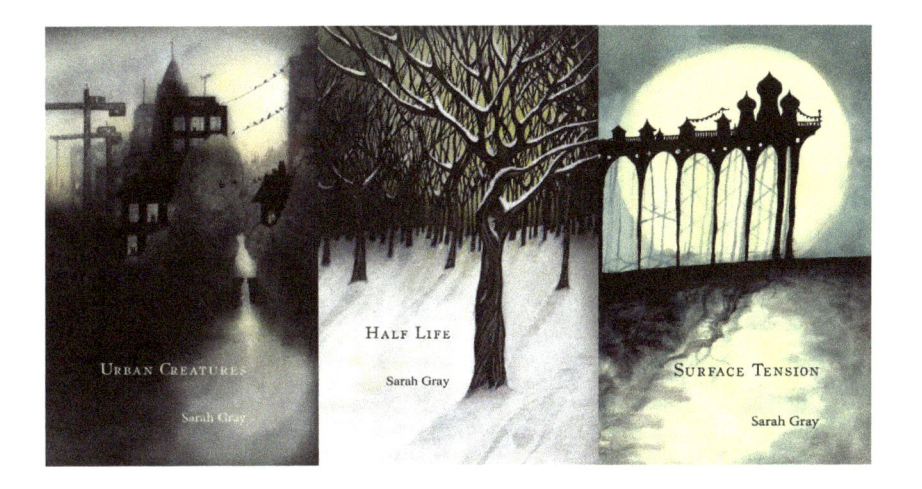